**ISBN:** 9781673609585

# EAT SMART

## U.S. Edition

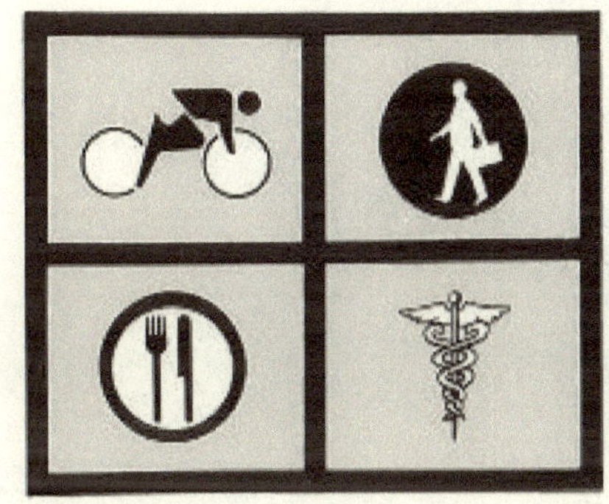

Gail Johnson, M.S.

**NoPaperPress**™

# CONTENTS

**TABLES**


**FIGURES**

## PREFACE

This eBook is intended for readers who want to improve their health by eating a more nutritious diet. Please note that *Eat Smart - U.S. Edition* is not only aimed at the "nutrition novice" but also at a person who has some understanding of nutrition but wants to learn more and go to the next level.

Because of the system of units employed in this edition (i.e., cups, pounds, etc), the book is intended primarily for United States residents. Readers in the remainder of the world would undoubtedly find *Eat Smart - Metric Edition* or *Eat Smart - U.K. Edition* easier to use and more beneficial.

Some of the material in this eBook was taken from *Weight Control - U.S. Edition* (with the permission of the author Vincent Antonetti, Ph.D.) an eBook and paperback also published by NoPaperPress.com.

Finally, I am indebted to my colleagues, former co-workers, nutritionists, friends, family and the NoPaperPress staff for their valuable suggestions and constructive criticism.

Gail Johnson

# 1. HEALTHY EATING IS VITAL

Despite all the nutrition-related books that populate libraries and bookstores, surveys indicate that very few people have a good understanding of nutrition and even fewer actually eat a healthy diet. When this is combined with a lack of exercise, it's no wonder that obesity is becoming a problem in many developed countries.

The physical conditions and living habits that increase the risk of premature heart disease, stroke and diabetes are well known, but there are counteracting step you can take. Said another way, to reduce your risk you need to look at your entire way of living and in some instances rearrange your priorities.

## Rules for a Healthy Life

No one set of rules will guarantee health. Age, gender, and physical condition are all factors in determining the specific program that is best for you. We can delineate, however, the general guidelines for a total health program:
- Have periodic medical checkups.
- Do not smoke.
- Practice good nutritional habits.
- Exercise regularly.
- Maintain a proper weight level.
- Learn to relax.
- Drink alcoholic in moderation.

This eBook concentrates on "Practice good nutritional habits."

## For Nutrition Professionals

Nutritionists, medical personnel, health education specialists, personal fitness trainers, and corporate fitness directors should find the data in this eBook useful in devising or supervising nutrition programs. Whether this book is used as a professional reference, or as a personal nutrition guide, our aim is to provide the nutrition facts and data needed for better health.

# Note that the material in this book is not intended as a substitute for medical counseling. Everyone should have a medical checkup before making major changes to their eating patterns. This is particularly important for anyone with medical problems and for women who are pregnant or breast- feeding, all of whom should consult a physician or registered dietician to determine the dietary pattern that is appropriate for them.

# 2. HOW HEALTHY ARE YOU?

Stated or not, everyone has goals in mind when they decide to consume more nutritious foods. It could be improving your health, reducing your risk of illness, lowering your blood cholesterol numbers, improving your appearance, or losing weight. Before you embark on a nutritional program and change your eating habits, however, you should know where you stand, i.e., your current health level. Assessing your status will help you establish what you should emphasize in your nutritional program and help you set goals.

## See Your Doctor First

In our opinion, everyone should have a medical checkup before starting a new nutritional program. The medical checkup may be as simple as a visit to a physician who is familiar with your medical history, or it may be a thorough physical exam.

Note, in all cases the physician conducting the medical exam should be made aware of and should approve the specific program you're planning. Besides a clinical exam by the physician, your medical exam will probably involve a blood chemistry test to determine your total, LDL and HDL cholesterol, triglycerides, blood glucose level, etcetera, and depending on your age and medical history may require a resting or exercising EKG.

## Body-Weight Self Assessment

Most people want to know what their body weight should be. In 1943, the Metropolitan Life Insurance Company introduced Weight versus Height tables for men and women. (MetLife published revised Weight versus Height tables in 1983.) The tables list weights associated with people who had the lowest mortality rates (lived the longest). The Met Life table yields reasonable weights for women who are slightly shorter than the average height, but the listed weights are not applicable to very short people, and the table lists impossibly low weights for tall women. The tables were also intended for adults ages 25 to 59 years. Their applicability to younger and older adults is problematic. And the MetLife tables would not be appropriate for competitive athletes, body builders, women who are pregnant or breast-feeding and the chronically ill.

## BMI-Based Weight vs. Height

More recently, many health-care practitioners rely on Body Mass Index, or BMI, to determine if a person is overweight. The BMI takes into account both a person's weight and height and is calculated by dividing a person's weight in kilograms by the square of their height (in meters). For United States readers, Table 1 provides a convenient determination of BMI, using body weight in pounds and height in feet and inches.  Again, this table would not be applicable to competitive athletes, body builders, women who are pregnant or breast-feeding and the chronically ill.

| Weight (lbs.) | - Height - | | | | | | | | | |
|---|---|---|---|---|---|---|---|---|---|---|
| | 60" | 62" | 64" | 66" | 68" | 70" | 72" | 74" | 76" | 78" |
| 100 | 19.6 | 18.3 | | | | | | | | |
| 110 | 21.5 | 20.1 | 18.9 | 17.8 | | | | | | |
| 120 | 23.5 | 22.0 | 20.6 | 19.4 | 18.3 | | | | | |
| 140 | 27.4 | 25.6 | 24.0 | 22.6 | 21.3 | 20.1 | 19.0 | | | |
| 160 | 31.3 | 29.3 | 27.5 | 25.8 | 24.3 | 23.0 | 21.7 | 20.6 | 19.5 | |
| 180 | 35.2 | 33.0 | 30.9 | 29.0 | 27.4 | 25.8 | 24.4 | 23.1 | 21.9 | 20.8 |
| 200 | 39.1 | 36.6 | 34.3 | 32.3 | 30.4 | 28.7 | 27.1 | 25.7 | 24.3 | 23.1 |
| 220 | 43.0 | 40.3 | 37.8 | 35.5 | 33.4 | 31.3 | 29.8 | 28.2 | 26.8 | 25.4 |
| 240 | 46.9 | 43.9 | 41.2 | 38.7 | 36.5 | 34.4 | 32.6 | 30.8 | 29.2 | 27.8 |
| 260 | 50.8 | 47.6 | 44.7 | 42.0 | 39.5 | 37.3 | 35.3 | 33.4 | 31.6 | 30.1 |
| 280 | | 51.3 | 48.1 | 45.2 | 42.6 | 40.2 | 38.0 | 35.9 | 34.1 | 32.4 |
| 300 | | | 51.5 | 48.5 | 45.6 | 43.0 | 40.7 | 38.6 | 36.5 | 34.7 |
| 400 | | | | | | | 54.3 | 51.4 | 48.7 | 46.3 |

**Table 1  Body Mass Index (BMI)**

| BMI | Weight Profile |
|---|---|
| 18.5 or less | Underweight |
| 18.6 to 24.9 | Normal |
| 25.0 to 29.9 | Overweight |
| 30.0 to 39.9 | Obese |
| 40 or more | Extremely Obese |

**Table 2  Weight Profile vs. BMI**

The rationale behind the BMI is based on epidemiological data that show an increase in mortality when the BMI is above 25, although the increase in mortality tends to be moderate until a BMI of 30 is reached.  Table 2 shows how a person's body-weight is categorized as a function of their BMI.

Another more convenient way to use BMI is the **New** BMI-Based Weight vs. Height Chart shown in Table 3, where the underweight category corresponds to BMI = 18.5 or less, normal weight is for BMI = 18.6 to 24.9, overweight is for BMI = 25.0 to 29.9, obese is for BMI = 30.0 to 39.9 and extremely obese is for BMI = 40 or more.  Note that the underweight and extremely obese categories are not shown in Table 3.

### Table 3  BMI-Based Weight vs. Height

| Height | Normal | Overweight | Obese |
|---|---|---|---|
| 4' 10" | 90 – 119 | 120 – 142 | 143 – 191 |
| 4' 11" | 93 – 123 | 124 – 148 | 149 – 197 |
| 5' 0" | 96 – 127 | 128 – 152 | 153 – 204 |
| 5' 1" | 99 – 131 | 132 – 158 | 159 – 211 |
| 5' 2" | 102 – 135 | 136 – 163 | 164 – 218 |
| 5' 3" | 105 – 140 | 141 – 169 | 170 – 225 |
| 5' 4" | 109 – 144 | 145 – 173 | 174 – 232 |
| 5' 5" | 112 – 149 | 150 – 180 | 181 – 239 |
| 5' 6" | 116 – 154 | 155 – 185 | 186 – 247 |
| 5' 7" | 119 – 159 | 160 – 191 | 192 – 254 |
| 5' 8" | 123 – 163 | 164 – 196 | 197 – 262 |
| 5' 9" | 126 – 168 | 169 – 202 | 203–270 |
| 5' 10" | 130 – 173 | 174 – 206 | 207 – 278 |
| 5' 11" | 134 – 178 | 179 – 214 | 215 – 286 |
| 6' 0" | 137 – 183 | 184 – 220 | 221 – 294 |
| 6' 1" | 141 – 188 | 189 – 227 | 228 – 302 |
| 6' 2" | 145 – 194 | 195 – 232 | 233 – 310 |
| 6' 3" | 149 – 199 | 200 – 239 | 240 – 319 |
| 6' 4" | 152 – 205 | 206 - 246 | 247 - 328 |
| 6' 5" | 157 - 210 | 211 - 252 | 253 – 337 |
| 6' 6" | 161 - 216 | 217 - 259 | 260 - 346 |

<u>**Example**</u>:  Determine BMI of a 5' 6" woman who weighs 160 pounds.  First use Table 1.  Scan the far left of the table and locate her weight of 160 pounds.  From this number run your finger horizontally (to the right) until it intersects the vertical column headed by her 5' 6" height.  The number at the

intersection is her BMI = 25.8.  According to Table 2 she is slightly overweight.

**Example**:  Determine the "normal" (healthy) weight for a man who is 6' 2" tall.  From Table 3, find that at 6' 2" this man must weigh between 145 and 194 pounds for his weight to be in the "normal" range, that is for his BMI to be between 18.6 and 24.9.  I think you will agree that the weight ranges provided by Table 3 are more useful than the BMI number from Table 1.

**Waist-to-Hip Ratio:**  Another important weight-profile parameter is your waist-to-hip ratio.  Health risks for heart attack and stroke increase considerably for:
  - Men with a waist to hip ratio greater than 1.0.
  - Women with a waist to hip ratio greater than 0.8.
To calculate your ratio, measure your waist size (at its narrowest circumference) and divide it by your hip size (at the widest section).  For example, a man with a 44 inch waist and 36 inch hips would have a waist to hip ratio of 42 / 36 = 1.2, and would have an increased risk for a heart attack or stroke.

## Are You Eating Sensibly?

To broadly assess how appropriate your current nutritional practices are please complete the following questionnaire.  (You may need pencil and paper to keep your score.)

**a) Number of vegetable servings eaten per day?**
  None (1 point)
  1 serving (2 points)
  2 to 4 (3 points)
  5 or more (4 points)

**b) How many fruit servings do you eat in a day?**
  None (1 point)
  1 serving (2 points)
  2 to 4 (3 points)
  5 or more (4 points)

**c) Cereal & whole-grain bread servings in a day?**
  None (1 pt)
  1 serving (2 pts)
  2 to 4 (3 pts)
  5 or more (4 pts)

**d) How many times per week do you eat a fish or poultry?**
  Never (1 pt)
  1 time (2 pts)

2 to 3 (3 pts)
4 or more (4 pts)
**e) How do you prepare and eat poultry?**
Fry dark meat with skin & gravy (1 pt)
Bake or broil dark meat with skin & gravy (2 pts)
Bake or broil dark meat without skin (3 pts)

Bake or broil white meat without skin (4 pts)
**f) How many times per week do you eat beans, lentils, peas?**
Never (1 pt)
1 time (2 pts)
2 to 3 (3 pts)
4 or more (4 pts)
**g) How often per week do you eat hamburger, salami, frankfurter, bacon, etc?**
7 or more (1 pt)
4 to 6 (2 pts)
2 to 3 (3 pts)
Rarely (4 pts)
**h) When you consume milk, yogurt, ice cream, etc, you most often select:**
Only whole-fat dairy product (1 pt)
Whole milk, but low-fat yogurt and ice cream (2 pts)
Low-fat (1 or 2% fat) (3 pts)
Skim or non-fat products (4 pts)
**i) If ordering potatoes in a restaurant would you choose:**
French fried or hash brown (1 pt)
Baked or boiled with butter and/or sour cream (2 pts)
Boiled without butter or sour cream (3 pts)
Baked without butter or sour cream (4 pts)
**j) How many times per week do you eat fast-food?**
5 or more (1 pt)
3 or 4 times (2 pts)
1 or 2 (3 pts)
Rarely (4 pts)
**k) Do you add salt to your food?**
At every meal (1 pt)l
Once per day (2 pts)
2 or 3 times per week (3 pts)
Rarely (4 pts)
**l) Do you eat sweets (cookies, candy bar, etc)?**
More than one sweet per day (1 pt)

About one per day (2 pts)
2 to 4 sweets per week (3 pts)
Rarely (4 pts)
**m) Do you take any vitamin or mineral supplements?**
None (1 pt)
Take herbal supplements (2 pts)
Take individual vitamins (like C, E, etc) (3 pts)

Take multi-vitamin and mineral supplement (4 pts)
**n) If you want to lose weight, how do you proceed?**
Go on a crash die (1 pt)
Stop eating carbs (2 pts)
Cut back on carbs & increase exercise (3 pts)
Reduce caloric intake & increase exercise (4 pts)
This completes our brief nutrition practices assessment.  Add up your score and see how you compare to the following standards.
Excellent = 49 to 56 points
Good =  41 to 48
Fair =  32 to 40
Poor =  23 to 31
Very Poor = 14 to 22

## Time to Set Goals
Now it's time to review your medical exam and self-assessment test results and set some broad personal goals, such lowering your LDL cholesterol. You're not quite ready to construct a total program.  That will have to wait until you read the in-depth chapters that follow.

# 3. NUTRITION FUNDAMENTALS

In the opinion of many researchers the makeup of the diet eaten by the majority of people in the United States is the single most important factor, albeit not the only one, accounting for our high incidence of overweight, and of death from coronary heart disease and stroke. It's no coincidence that accompanying the high mortality numbers is an increase in the amount of fat we eat, an increase in the number of calories consumed per capita, and the inevitable increase in the average weight of our citizens. All are directly attributable to our diet.

Mistaken notions about nutrition point out how little understanding many of us have about what our bodies need for energy and repair. Often we eat what's easiest to prepare, what's tastiest, or what's at hand – without thinking about nutritional content or giving much thought to the eventual consequences. It's a scientific fact that prolonged poor nutrition is a definite threat to your health.

In this chapter you will learn how to improve the "nutritional quality" of the food you eat, and, as expected, we will also point out foods that you should avoid, i.e., "junk" foods, those foods that are loaded with "nutritionally-empty calories."

## "Junk" Foods on the Increase

Nutritionists and consumer advocates are increasingly concerned that often enjoyable but nutritionally deficient foods, i.e., "junk" foods, are finding to large a place in the American diet. What is a "junk" food? A nutritionist defines a "junk" food as one that offers little if any essential nutrients – except calories – and is used to replace more important foods. Often "junk" foods are snack foods, "fun" foods and are being used more and more by the consumer as meal replacements.

## Confusion in Supermarkets

Supermarkets have all the foods you need – and in abundance. But humans are not designed to resist food. Just the opposite. From pre-historic times, we are genetically programmed to eat when food is available – and eat we do!

Most shoppers are bewildered by the vast array of food choices in our supermarkets. Many foods can be purchased fresh, frozen, dehydrated, concentrated, etcetera; then there are special diet foods, ethnic foods, and on and on. Despite all these options, most nutritionists agree that a great many Americans are not eating well enough to sustain good health. In general, our diet is too high in fat – with an average of 40 percent of our calories from fat – contributing to atherosclerosis.

Another culprit is sugar. As a nation we consume more than 100 pounds of sugar per year per person, totaling an unhealthy, nutritionally empty, 500 Calories per day. This large intake of sugar leads to obvious ills, such as obesity and tooth decay.

Add to this the increased use of processed and convenience foods, the proliferation of nutritional misinformation and deceptive advertising, and it is clear that you must improve your understanding of nutrition in order to eat properly.

## Your Metabolic Pathways

Early men and women evolved a storage system for survival during alternating periods of plenty and fasting. Physiologists describe these two functional periods as the absorptive state, when the food we eat enters the blood and lymph from the gastrointestinal tract (GI tract), and the post-absorptive stage, or fasting state, when the GI tract is empty and energy is supplied by the body's energy storage system – the body's adipose tissue, or fat.

During the absorptive period diagramed in Figure 1, fat droplets (triglycerides) are absorbed directly into the lymph and stored in the adipose tissue. Carbohydrates (primarily in the form of glucose) and protein (amino acids) enter the blood stream. All the blood leaving the GI tract goes to the liver.

Although glucose is the body's major energy source during the absorptive state, much of the glucose is converted in the liver to glycogen and stored as an immediately available energy source. A small fraction, of the amino acids in the food you eat, is used for energy; another fraction is used to resynthesize continuously degrading body tissue. Any excess calories, whether carbohydrate, protein, or fat, are stored in the adipose tissue as fat.

During the post-absorptive period illustrated in Figure 2, when there is no food in the GI tract, the essential problem is that the blood glucose level must be maintained for the survival of the brain and nervous system, which can only use glucose as an energy source. If your blood sugar (glucose) level falls too low you become dizzy and feel faint. Glycogen stores are your first line of defense, and supply your body's glucose needs for several hours when your GI tract is empty – pointing out the importance of carbohydrates in the diet. If fasting continues, protein and to a lesser extent fat are used to produce the glucose needed by the nervous system. Meanwhile, the other organs and tissues of the body go into a glucose-sparing mode and utilize fat as an energy source.

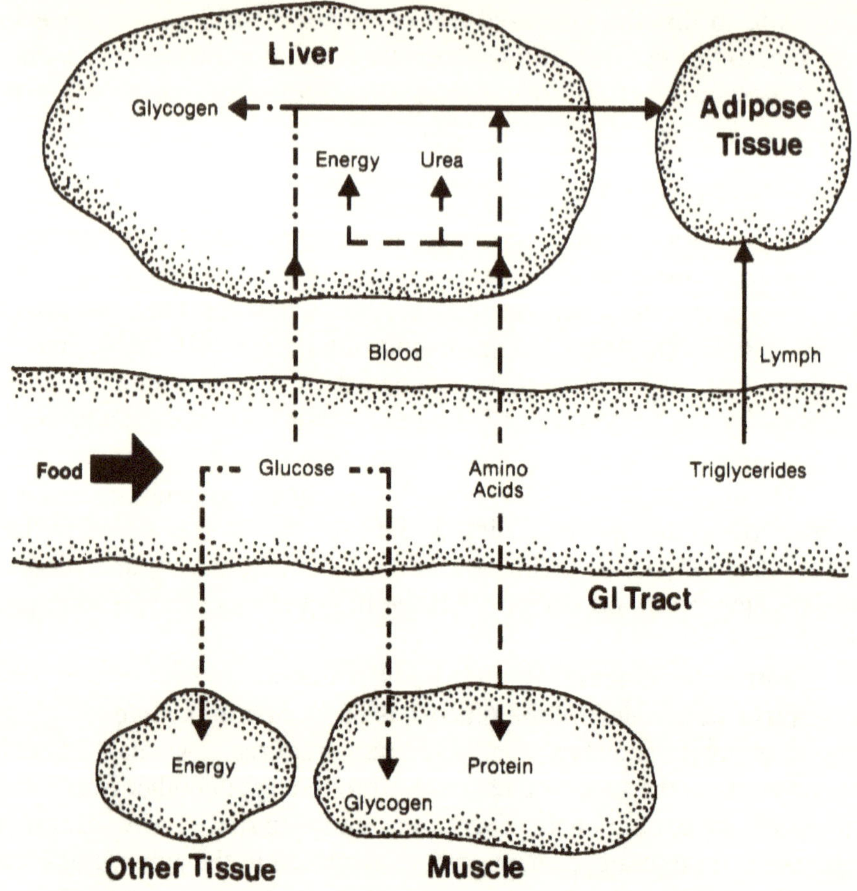


**Figure 1:  Metabolic Pathways - Absorptive Stage**

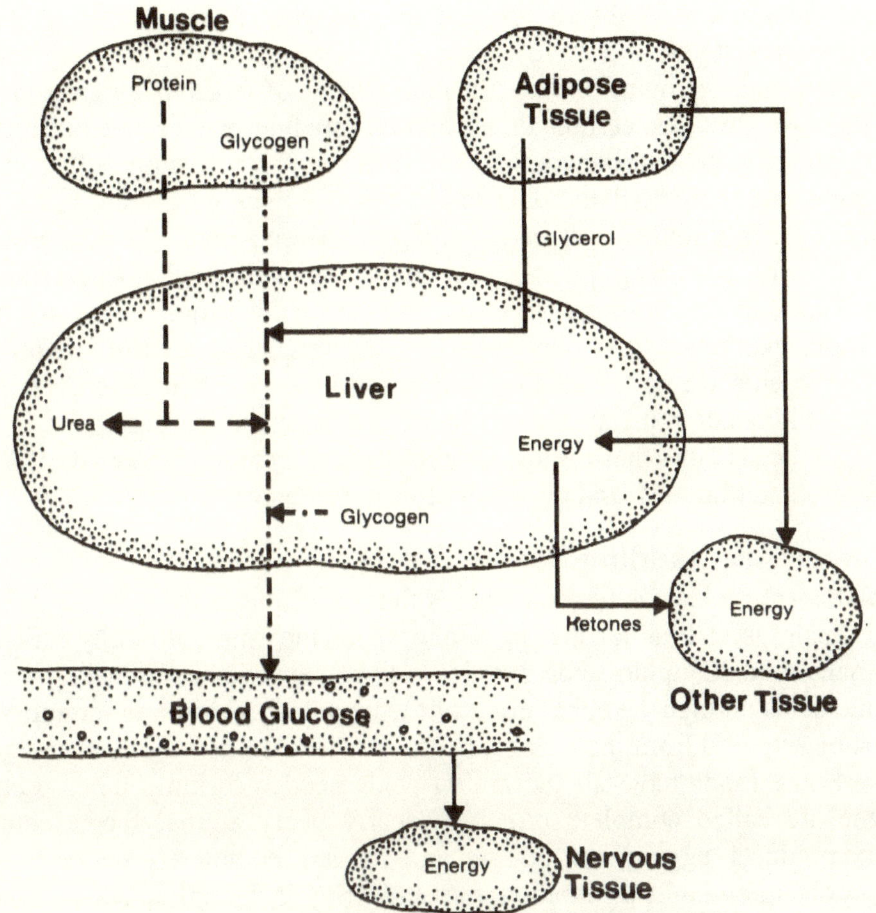


**Figure 2: Metabolic Pathways - Post-Absorptive**

Our bodies are renewed by what we eat. And food should give us pleasure as well as nourishment. Good nutritional practices can not only be rewarding be also be fun to learn about and to put into practice. And feeling and seeing the results of good nutrition can not only be a source of satisfaction, but also can be the motivation you need to tackle other phases of a total health program — such as starting an exercise program or giving up cigarettes.

## Nutrients & Micronutrients

Foods are made up of seven basic constituents: carbohydrates, proteins, fats, vitamins, minerals, fiber and water. For a healthy body you need to eat the correct quantity and proportion of all these components. You need protein, carbohydrates and fats, for growth, repair and energy. You need vitamins and minerals, albeit in relatively small quantities, so they can perform their

17

vital roles in the thousands of biochemical reactions in your body. Fiber, the broad name given to the things you eat that your bodies cannot digest, is needed to assist your digestive system

Nutrients and micronutrients are the components of foods that are essential to human life. Proteins, carbohydrates and fats are nutrients. Some nutritionists refer to proteins, carbohydrates and fats as "macronutrients," and call vitamins and minerals "micronutrients" because they are present in foods in much smaller amounts than macronutrients. More recently, a new grouping of naturally occurring plant-based chemicals, called phytochemicals, or phytonutrients by some nutritionists, have been identified as having many healthful qualities, but unlike traditional macronutrients and micronutrients, phytonutrients are not needed by humans to live; i.e., their absence will not necessarily result in metabolic problems, or a deficiency disease.

In the sections that follow we will discuss proteins, carbohydrates, fats, vitamins and minerals, and phytonutrients in some detail.

## Proteins are Building Blocks

Proteins are molecules of amino acids that are required for cell maintenance and repair, as well as for the regulation of a wide range of bodily functions. Humans need 22 amino acids in order to live. Our bodies can make 14 of the amino acids on their own, but eight of them, called the essential-amino acids, must be acquired from the foods we eat.

Some foods have all the amino acids needed to build other proteins. These are called complete proteins. Nearly every animal food, including dairy products, eggs, meat, poultry and fish are complete proteins because they contain all eight-essential amino acids. Soy is the only plant-based food that has all eight essential-amino acids.

Other plant-based protein sources lack one or more essential amino acids (i.e., amino acids that the body can't either create, or manufacture by modifying other amino acids.) These incomplete proteins are found in legumes, grains, nuts, and seeds. However, consuming combinations of foods that have incomplete proteins can provide the same complete protein end effect as animal protein.

**For a complete-protein meal, simply eat any of the incomplete proteins with another but different incomplete protein.** Examples of some healthy plant-protein combinations (that provide complete protein) are:

<u>**Eating grains with legumes:**</u> pasta and beans, rice and lentils, tortillas with refried beans, etc

<u>**Eating grains with nuts or seeds:**</u> peanut butter on whole-grain bread, etc

Around the world, millions of people don't get enough protein.  Protein malnutrition can cause growth failure, loss of muscle mass, decreased immunity, weakening of the heart and respiratory system, and in some cases death.  Whereas, in the United States and other developed countries, getting the minimum daily requirement of protein is usually not a problem, because almost any reasonable diet will provide most of us with sufficient protein.

Adults need about 0.79 grams of protein for every kilogram of body weight per day to keep from slowly breaking down their own tissue.  **(This translates as approximately 0.36 grams of protein for every pound of body weight.)**  A case in point, an adult weighing 154 pounds (70 kg) requires about (154 x 0.36), or 55 grams of protein per day.  How much protein is in food?  A few examples:  There are approximately seven grams of protein per ounce of beef, poultry, fish, cheese or peanuts. Soybeans pack 10 grams of protein per ounce.  Most other beans and lentils contain about six grams of protein per ounce.  There are roughly three grams of protein in an ounce of whole-grain cereal, and milk has one gram of protein per fluid ounce.

Understand that foods are rarely straight protein.  Some high-protein foods, such as marbled beef and whole milk, also come with lots of unhealthy saturated fat.  Therefore, when you eat meat, eat the leanest cuts, and when you consume dairy products, choose skim or low-fat varieties. On the other hand, beans, nuts, and whole grains offer protein with little saturated fat – but with lots of healthful fiber and micronutrients.

## You Need the Right Carbs

Carbohydrates provide your body with its basic fuel, the energy your cells need to survive.  The staple of most diets around the world, carbohydrates provide essential vitamins and minerals, fiber, and numerous beneficial compounds (phytonutrients) that promote good health.

The simplest carbohydrate is glucose. Also called "blood sugar" and "dextrose," glucose flows in the bloodstream so that it is available to every cell in your body.  Your body's cells absorb glucose and convert it into energy to drive the cell.  Glucose is a simple sugar, meaning that it tastes sweet. Some other simple sugars are sucrose, also known as "white sugar," fructose, the main sugar in fruits, and lactose, the sugar found in milk.  They all taste sweet, and most are digested and enter your bloodstream quickly. When you eat fruit or drink milk, however, the natural sugar comes with vitamins, minerals (as well as fiber when you eat fruit); whereas the simple sugars in candy, for instance, are nothing but nutritionally-empty calories.

Then there are the more complex carbohydrates.  Most grains (wheat, corn, oats, rice) and foods like potatoes, pasta and plantains are complex carbohydrates.   In general, but not always, complex carbohydrates are digested more slowly than simple carbohydrates, and take much longer to enter your bloodstream.   Most of us have heard that eating complex carbohydrates is good, and eating sugar-loaded foods is a bad.  The reason is that simple sugars require little digestion, and when you eat a sweet food, such as a candy bar, or drink a can of soda, your blood glucose level rises rapidly. In response, your pancreas secretes a large amount of insulin to keep your blood glucose levels from rising too high.  The large insulin response in turn tends to cause your blood sugar to fall to levels that are too low.  As a consequence, about three to five hours after consuming sweets you feel lethargic and hungry.  Many people react to this by eating yet another sweet, which can start a rollercoaster ride of surging glucose and then insulin.  None of this is experienced after eating most complex carbohydrates, or a balanced meal, because the digestion and absorption processes are much slower.

## Glycemic Index Defined

Thinking of carbohydrates as complex or simple, as good or bad, is outdated. More recently, a system has been devised to classify carbohydrates.  The system, called the glycemic index (GI), measures the effect a carbohydrate has on your blood sugar – quantifying how rapidly and to what level your blood sugar rises after you eat a food containing carbohydrates, compared to a reference food (usually glucose or white bread).  For instance, a candy bar, which is digested rapidly has a high GI and causes an almost immediate jump in your blood sugar; whereas, lentil soup is digested more slowly and has a low GI.  The factors that influence a food's GI are:

**1) Fiber** prevents the rapid digestion of the carbohydrates in food and slows the discharge of sugar molecules into the blood stream. Higher fiber content results in a lower GI.

**2) Coarsely-ground grains** are digested more slowly and, therefore, have lower GI values than finely-ground grains.

**3) Less-processed** carbohydrates, such whole-grain foods where the fiber, bran and germ are intact, are digested more slowly than highly-processed carbohydrates.  In general, therefore, less processing usually results in a lower GI.

**4) Unripe** fruits and vegetables contain less sugar and have a lower GI than ripe varieties.

**5) The more acid or fat** a food has, the slower its carbohydrates are digested and absorbed into the blood stream.  More acid and fat in a food mean a lower GI.

These factors sometimes lead to unexpected results.  For instance, some foods containing simple carbohydrates such as fruit have a lower GI than a complex carbohydrate like the potato.

The glycemic index uses a scale of 0 to 100, with foods that cause the most rapid rise in blood sugar having the highest values.  In this book and many others, glucose is the arbitrary reference food, and is assigned a GI = 100.  (For a given food, a GI less than 56 is considered low, a GI = 56 to 69 is medium, and a GI greater than 69 is high.)  Note that foods that contain little or no carbohydrate (such as meat, fish, eggs, avocado, wine, beer and other alcoholic beverages) do not have GI values.

## Glycemic Load - More Meaning

Some food scientists have come to recognize that a food's GI value alone does not provide enough information to judge how a particular food will affect your blood sugar.  This is because the GI does not take into account how much carbohydrate is in a food serving, and your blood sugar level is influenced by both the quality of the carbohydrate (GI) and the quantity of carbohydrate you eat.  With this in mind, researchers developed a new guideline called the glycemic load (GL) which takes into account both a food's GI and the quantity of carbohydrate the food contains.  A food's GL is calculated by multiplying the food's GI by the number of carbohydrate grams in a serving.  For a given food, a GL less 11 is considered low, a GL = 11 to 19 is medium, and a GL greater than 19 is high.  Most people consume 60 to 180 GL units per day, with a total GL of about 100 for a typical diet.

Table 3 presents GI and GL values for some common foods.  Most of the data are from the on-line database of the University of Sidney (Australia). The difference between a food's GI and GL is illustrated by a simple example.  Watermelon (not shown in Table 3) has a GI = 72, quite high.  In this case, however, GI alone is misleading because watermelon only has about six grams of carbohydrate per serving.  (Watermelon is almost entirely water, with some fiber and a small quantity of carbohydrate.)  So a typical serving of watermelon, has a GL = GI x (net carb grams) = 0.72 x 6 = 4.3, which is quite low.  (Note in the calculation, watermelon's GI value has been converted from 72% to the decimal equivalent 0.72.)

| Food | Glycemic Index (%) | Serving Size | Net Carbs | Glycemic Load |
| --- | --- | --- | --- | --- |
| Strawberries | 40 | 1 cup (150 g) | 3 | 1 |
| Peanuts | 14 | 3.5 oz. (100 g) | 9 | 1 |
| Peach | 42 | large (120 g) | 8 | 3 |
| Carrot | 92 | large (80 g) | 4 | 4 |
| Lentils | 28 | 1 cup (150 g) | 15 | 4 |
| Orange | 48 | medium (120 g) | 9 | 4 |
| Watermelon | 72 | 1 cup (120 g) | 6 | 4 |
| Apple | 40 | medium (138 g) | 15 | 6 |
| Ice Cream | 65 | 1 scoop (50 g) | 10 | 7 |
| Bread (wheat) | 73 | 1 slice (30 g) | 11 | 8 |
| Grapes | 46 | 4 oz. (120 g) | 18 | 8 |
| Bread (white) | 70 | 1 slice (30 g) | 13 | 9 |
| Corn (sweet) | 59 | 1 ear (80 g) | 16 | 9 |
| Banana | 50 | large (120 g) | 24 | 12 |
| Oatmeal | 58 | 1 cup (234 g) | 21 | 12 |
| Sweet potato | 50 | medium (150 g) | 26 | 13 |
| Spaghetti | 45 | 6 oz. (180 g) | 44 | 20 |
| Potato (baked) | 94 | medium (150 g) | 22 | 21 |
| Rice (brown) | 50 | 4.5 oz. (130 g) | 48 | 24 |
| Raisins | 64 | 1 box (60 g) | 43 | 28 |
| Rice (white) | 72 | 4.5 oz. (130 g) | 42 | 30 |
| Snickers candy | 55 | 1 bar (113 g) | 64 | 35 |
| Glucose | 100 | (50 g) | 50 | 50 |

**Table 4:  Glycemic Rank of Common Foods**

Some diet book authors claim a food's GI and in some cases GL are the most important guidelines to use when planning a weight-loss diet.  But consider the following:  Pears (not shown in Table 3) are forbidden by some diets because of a relatively high GI = 40.  However, a medium size pear weighing about four ounces has a GL = 4, quite low.  Now consider a four ounce serving of peanuts with a much lower GI = 14, and an even lower GL = 2. For people on a reducing diet, based only on Glycemic Index or Load, a snack of peanuts appears to be a better choice than a pear.  A medium-size pear, however, contains only 70 Calories, while four ounces  of peanuts are loaded with about 650 Calories!  Pears and peanuts are both healthy foods, but the extra 580 Calories in peanuts are certainly not going to help you lose weight.

The focus on a food's GI can lead to limiting healthful foods that may have a high GI by themselves, but when eaten in combination with other foods are not a problem.  A nutritious baked potato may have a high GI, but when eaten as part of a complete meal is digested more slowly than its GI value would indicate.  The main point is that if you use GI or GL values as the sole factor when selecting your food, you could be eliminating very healthy foods, and eating too many calories and often too much fat as well.  It is important, therefore, to appreciate that a food's GI and GL numbers only allow you to evaluate how a food's carbohydrate content affects your blood sugar level.  Because our body performs better when our blood sugar remains relatively constant, we should be aware of a food's GL rank and consider it when planning our eating pattern.  But there are other important factors that must also be taken into account, such as getting the micronutrients we need from a variety of foods, including carbohydrates, and staying within our caloric allowance.

In summary, **carbohydrates are neither all good nor all bad.** Remember good carbohydrates provide needed micronutrients.  You should try to get the bulk of your calories from the good carbohydrates, i.e., from fruits, from vegetables and from whole grains such as whole-grain cereal, whole-wheat bread, whole-grain pasta, whole-old-fashioned oats, brown rice, bulgur, millet, and hulled barley.

## Cholesterol and Triglycerides

Atherosclerosis has been linked to both blood cholesterol and triglyceride levels.  Both fatty substances are found in the plaque on the walls of clogged arteries. There are two types of cholesterol: high-density cholesterol (HDL), the "good" cholesterol, and low-density cholesterol (LDL), the "bad" cholesterol.  You should have your cholesterol and triglyceride levels measured during a regular medical checkup and should know and understand the readings.  At this writing, the desirable readings for otherwise healthy individuals are as follows:

- **Total cholesterol:  less than 200 mg/dl.**
- **HDL cholesterol:  greater than 40 mg/dl.**
- **LDL cholesterol:  less than 130 mg/dl.**
- **Triglycerides:  less than 150 mg/dl.**

For people who have coronary-artery disease, most cardiologists insist that the total cholesterol level be less than 160 mg/dl and the even more important LDL cholesterol be less than 100 mg/dl. Lately, cardiologists have been urging patients with coronary-artery disease to reduce their LDL even further to below 70 mg/dl.

Often, cholesterol and triglyceride levels can be reduced by adhering to the eating recommendations summarized at the end of the section that immediately follows, called "Fats in Foods." Where a low-fat diet alone does not work, people with high cholesterol and or high triglyceride levels, may be prescribed cholesterol-lowering medication by their physician. For more information on this important subject, visit the American Heart Association website: http://www.americanheart.org.

## The Skinny on Fat

Fats are found in vegetable oil, seeds and nuts, meat and fish, and dairy products, as well as in foods like potato chips and french fries (that are cooked in oil), cookies, cake, and so on. There are certain fats you absolutely need to survive (the essential-fatty acids), and others you would do well to drastically limit (saturated fats) or avoid altogether (trans fats). Chemically, all fatty acids contain carbon chains with hydrogen atoms bonded to the carbon, and all fats have the highest calorie density – containing nine calories per gram.

Until recently, the best wisdom was to eat a low-fat, low-cholesterol diet. This advice is now largely out of date. The latest research seems to show that the total amount of fat in the diet may not be strongly linked with disease. **What appears to matter is the type of fat in your diet.**

<u>Saturated Fats</u>: When all carbon bonds of a fat molecule are filled with hydrogen, a fat is said to be saturated, i.e., saturated with hydrogen atoms. Most saturated fats are animal in origin and are solid at room temperature (good examples are butter and the fat in meats). Generally speaking, you should avoid or at least severely limit your intake of saturated fats because they can raise both your total and bad LDL blood cholesterol levels which increases your chances of getting heart disease.

When hydrogen atoms are missing along the carbon chain the fatty acids are called monounsaturated or polyunsaturated depending on their exact chemical structure.

<u>Monounsaturated fats</u> (also called omega-9 fatty acids) are liquid at room temperature and are known as oils. They are "good fats" and are derived from plant sources, such as vegetable oils, nuts, and seeds. In studies in which monounsaturated fats were eaten in place of carbohydrates, LDL blood cholesterol levels decreased and HDL cholesterol levels increased. Monounsaturated fats are found in high concentrations in canola, olive and peanut oils.

24

**Polyunsaturated fats** are also liquid oils at room temperature and in your refrigerator. They are "good fats" and are derived from plant sources, such as vegetable oils, nuts, and seeds. Again, research has demonstrated that when polyunsaturated fats were eaten in place of carbohydrates, LDL blood cholesterol levels decreased and HDL cholesterol levels increased. Polyunsaturated fats are found in high concentrations in sunflower, soybean and corn oils.

- Essential-Fatty Acids are class of polyunsaturated fatty acids that our body cannot create. These fats must be obtained from the food you eat. Essential-fatty acids promote absorption of the fat-soluble vitamins A, D, E, and K and are also thought to provide many disease-fighting benefits. Because essential-fatty acids are needed and our body cannot manufacture them, they must come from the food we eat. Essential-fatty acids fall into two groups: omega-3 and omega-6.

- Omega-3 fatty acids are relatively hard to find. Foods high in omega-3 fatty acids are walnuts, tofu, flax seeds and oily fish (salmon, mackerel, sardines, trout and albacore tuna). Omega-3 fats are thought to be heart-protective. (The American Heart Association suggests that people with coronary-heart disease consult with their physician regarding the advisability of taking a fish-oil supplement.)

- Omega-6 fatty acids, on the other hand, are more common, easier to find, and are in most oils including sunflower, soybean and corn oils.

Current thinking is that the consumption of omega-6 and omega-3 fatty acids should be in the ratio of 3:1, with about three omega-6 for one omega-3. Many Western diets, however, contain about 15:1, omega-6 to omega-3, which is not good for your health. Although you need omega-6, people generally eat too much of it and not enough omega-3 fat. The American Heart Association recommends that you eat fish (particularly fatty fish) two times a week, as a way to get a more appropriate quantity of omega-3 fatty acids in your diet.

| Fat Type | Where found |
|---|---|
| **Saturated** | **Meat, poultry (especially the skin), dairy products, lard, coconut oil, palm oil, cocoa butter** |
| **Trans Fats** | **Fried foods, margarine, snack foods, commercially-baked cake and cookies, and fast foods** |
| **Cholesterol** | **Egg yokes, dairy products, organ meats, fatty and prime meats, poultry skin, shellfish (particularly shrimp)** |
| **Polyunsaturated (Omega-3)** | Mackerel, salmon, sardines, tuna, canola oil, walnuts, flaxseed, wheat germ |
| **Polyunsaturated (Omega-6)** | Corn oil, cottonseed oil, safflower oil, sunflower oil, soybean oil |
| **Monounsaturated (Omega-9)** | Canola oil, olive oil, safflower oil (hybrid), sunflower oil (hybrid) |

**Table 5:  Fats in Foods**

__Trans fats__ are produced when a liquid oil is processed into a solid fat.  The manufacturing process is called hydrogenation, or partial hydrogenation, and trans fats are an unnatural by-product.  Partially-hydrogenated vegetable oils are considered especially unhealthy, because of the resulting trans-fatty acids and the added hydrogen saturation.  Research indicates that trans fats are even worse than saturated fats because they not only raise bad LDL cholesterol but also  lower good HDL cholesterol.  Eliminating foods containing partially-hydrogenated oils from your diet is vital to good health.

**In summary**, it is becoming increasingly clear that saturated and trans fats, increase the risk for certain diseases while monounsaturated and polyunsaturated fats, lower the risk.  The key is not to eliminate fat from your diet but to substitute good fats for bad fats, and at the same time try to reduce the total amount of fat consumed because all fats are very high in calories.  The current scientific thinking regarding fat consumption is as follows:

**1)**  Try to limit the total fat you eat to no more than 30 percent of  your caloric intake.

**2)**  Do not consume foods containing partially-hydrogenated vegetable oil because they are high in trans fats.  This includes commercially prepared baked goods, snack foods, and processed foods, including fast foods.  To be on the safe-side, assume these food products contain trans fats unless labeled otherwise.

**3)** Limit saturated fats, i.e., any fat of animal origin, to 10 percent of your caloric intake. Have meat less often, and when serving meat use lean cuts and trim the fat. Eat fish and poultry (white meat, without the skin) more frequently. Use fat-free or low-fat-milk dairy products in place of whole-milk dairy products. (Coconut and palm oil should also be avoided because they are saturated fats.)

**4)** When consuming fat, choose foods containing monounsaturated fats like olive oil and canola oil, and foods rich in polyunsaturated omega-6 and omega-3 fatty acids.

**5)** Try to balance your intake essential fatty acids by eating more omega-3 fatty acids, found in walnuts, tofu, certain seeds and oily fish such as salmon, sardines and tuna.

## Vitamins and Minerals

The following is a listing of vitamins and minerals complete with a brief discussion of their function in your body, what foods supply the particular micronutrient, and the Recommended Dietary Allowance (RDA) - which is a reference number developed by the United States Food and Drug Administration to help consumers determine how much of a specific micronutrient a food contains. Summaries of the RDAs for vitamins and minerals are shown in Table 5a, 5b, 6a and Table 6b. Notice that RDAs are frequently gender and age dependent.

Because of the rapid expansion of scientific knowledge regarding the role of micronutrients in human health, the U.S. Food and Drug Administration, in partnership with Health Canada, periodically assesses and updates the recommended Daily Values. The following contains the recommended RDAs as of April 2006 for the vitamins and minerals discussed.

**Vitamin A** is a collection of fat-soluble compounds that play an important role in vision, bone growth, reproduction, cell division, and help prevent or fight off infections. Vitamin A also promotes healthy surface linings of the eyes, respiratory, urinary, and intestinal tracts, and also helps maintain the integrity of skin and mucous membranes. Using the long-established International Unit (IU) measure for the recommended dietary allowance (RDA), adult men and women need 3,000 and 2,330 IU (as retinol) per day respectively. However, the new RDA measure for vitamin A is the microgram (mcg), which translates for men and women as 900 and 700 mcg per day. Foods rich in vitamin A are orange-colored vegetables such as carrots, sweet potatoes and pumpkin; dark-green-leafy vegetables like spinach, collards and romaine lettuce; and orange-colored fruits such as mango, cantaloupe and apricots; and red peppers and tomatoes.  One medium-size carrot supplies approximately 270 percent of your RDA.

**Vitamin D** is a fat-soluble vitamin.  Briefly, vitamin D is important in assisting the absorption of calcium, in forming strong bones and teeth and preventing deficiency diseases such as rickets and osteomalacia.  For most adults, an adequate intake of vitamin D is 200 to 600 IU (which is equivalent to 5 to 15 mcg per day).  In addition, your body can make vitamin D after exposure to sunshine.  Good food sources include salt-water fish such as herring, salmon, sardines and fish-liver oils, as well as fortified milk and cereals.  Small quantities are also found in egg yokes, veal and beef.  An eight-ounce glass of fortified milk supplies about 25 percent of your daily needs.

**Vitamin E** is a fat-soluble vitamin that is a powerful antioxidant and acts to protect cells against the effects of free radicals.  Research is underway to determine if vitamin E, through its ability to limit the production of free radicals, might help prevent or delay the development of cardiovascular disease and some cancers.  For adults, the RDA for vitamin E is 22.5 IU (as d-alpha-tocopherol) which is equal to 15 mcg per day.  Foods rich in vitamin E are vegetable oils, nuts, seeds, milk fat, egg yolks, liver, dark-green-leafy vegetables, and whole-grain foods.  Approximately 12 almonds provide 100 percent of RDA for vitamin E.

| Vitamin | Ages | | | |
| --- | --- | --- | --- | --- |
| | 19-30 | 31-50 | 51-70 | 70+ |
| A (mcg) | 900 | 900 | 900 | 900 |
| D (mcg) | 5 | 5 | 10 | 15 |
| E (mcg) | 15 | 15 | 15 | 15 |
| K (mcg) | 120 | 120 | 120 | 120 |
| C (mg) | 90 | 90 | 90 | 90 |
| $B_1$ (mg) | 1.2 | 1.2 | 1.2 | 1.2 |
| $B_2$ (mg) | 1.3 | 1.3 | 1.3 | 1.3 |
| $B_3$ (mg) | 16 | 16 | 16 | 16 |
| $B_5$ (mg) | 5 | 5 | 5 | 5 |
| $B_6$ (mg) | 1.3 | 1.3 | 1.7 | 1.7 |
| $B_7$ (mcg) | 30 | 30 | 30 | 30 |
| $B_9$ (mcg) | 400 | 400 | 400 | 400 |
| $B_{12}$ (mcg) | 2.4 | 2.4 | 2.4 | 2.4 |

**Table 6a: Vitamin RDA for Men**

Values for vitamins D, K, $B_5$ and $B_7$ are Adequate Intake.  mcg = micrograms per day  mg = milligrams per day.

| Vitamin | Age | | | | | |
|---|---|---|---|---|---|---|
| | 19-30 | 31-50 | 51-70 | 70+ | Preg | Lact |
| **A** (mcg) | 700 | 700 | 700 | 700 | 770 | 1300 |
| **D** (mcg) | 5 | 5 | 10 | 15 | 5 | 5 |
| **E** (mcg) | 15 | 15 | 15 | 15 | 15 | 19 |
| **K** (mcg) | 90 | 90 | 90 | 90 | 90 | 90 |
| **C** (mg) | 75 | 75 | 75 | 75 | 85 | 120 |
| **$B_1$** (mg) | 1.1 | 1.1 | 1.1 | 1.1 | 1.4 | 1.4 |
| **$B_2$** (mg) | 1.1 | 1.1 | 1.1 | 1.1 | 1.4 | 1.6 |
| **$B_3$** (mg) | 14 | 14 | 14 | 14 | 18 | 17 |
| **$B_5$** (mg) | 5 | 5 | 5 | 5 | 6 | 7 |
| **$B_6$** (mg) | 1.3 | 1.3 | 1.5 | 1.5 | 1.9 | 2.0 |
| **$B_7$** (mcg) | 30 | 30 | 30 | 30 | 30 | 35 |
| **$B_9$** (mcg) | 400 | 400 | 400 | 400 | 600 | 500 |
| **$B_{12}$** (mcg) | 2.4 | 2.4 | 2.4 | 2.4 | 2.6 | 2.8 |

### Table 6b: Vitamin RDA for Women

Values for vitamins D, K, $B_5$ and $B_7$ are Adequate Intake.  Preg = pregnant  Lact = lactating mcg = micrograms per day  mg = milligrams per day.

**Vitamin K** is another fat-soluble vitamin, and is known as the clotting vitamin because without it blood would not clot. Some studies also indicate that it helps maintain strong bones in the elderly.  Adequate intake of vitamin K for men is 120 mcg per day and for women 90 mcg per day.  Food sources are dark-green-leafy vegetables, soybean, cottonseed, canola, and olive oil. People who eat these foods as part of a balanced diet should easily get enough vitamin K.

**Vitamin C** is a water-soluble, antioxidant vitamin.  It is important in forming collagen, a protein that gives structure to bones, cartilage, muscle, and blood vessels.  Vitamin C also aids in the absorption of iron, and helps maintain capillaries, bones, and teeth.   The RDA for vitamin C is 90 milligrams (mg) per day for men and 75 mg per day for women.  Foods rich in vitamin C are citrus fruits and juices, kiwifruit, strawberries, cantaloupe, broccoli, peppers, tomatoes, cabbage potatoes,  and  dark-green-leafy vegetables. A six-ounce glass of orange juice supplies 100 percent of a man's RDA.

**Vitamin B** is actually a complex of different water-soluble vitamins that often exist in the same foods. They perform an important role in our metabolism, in maintaining muscle tone along our digestive tract and in the health of our nervous system, skin, hair, eyes, mouth, and liver.  he B complex vitamins are: vitamin $B_1$ (thiamine), vitamin $B_2$ (riboflavin), vitamin $B_3$ (niacin), vitamin $B_5$ (pantothenic acid), vitamin $B_6$ (pyridoxine), vitamin $B_7$ (biotin), vitamin $B_9$ (folic acid), and vitamin $B_{12}$ (cyanocobalamin). Many cereals are fortified with all the B vitamins.  Depending on the brand, one serving of a fortified cereal provides from 25 to 100 percent of the RDA for all the B vitamins (except vitamin $B_7$ biotin).

**Vitamin $B_1$ (thiamine)** plays a vital role in the proper operation of your nervous system. Your body also needs $B_1$ to convert carbohydrates into sugar and then energy.  The RDA for men is 1.2 mg per day and 1.1 mg per day for women.  Vitamin $B_1$ is found in meat, wheat germ, whole-grains cereals and breads, in enriched cereals and breads, in beans, nuts and seeds, and in dark-green-leafy vegetables.

**Vitamin $B_2$ (riboflavin)** also has a crucial role in certain metabolic reactions, particularly the conversion of carbohydrates into energy. Riboflavin is also an important antioxidant.  he RDA is 1.3 mg per day for men and 1.1 mg per day for women.  he best sources of riboflavin are brewer's yeast, almonds, organ meats, whole grains, wheat germ, wild rice, mushrooms, soybeans, milk, yogurt, eggs, broccoli, and spinach.  In addition, flour and cereals are often fortified with riboflavin.

**Vitamin $B_3$ (niacin)** helps clear toxic and harmful chemicals from your body.  It also assists in the production of various hormones.  Niacin improves your circulation and reduces blood cholesterol levels.  The RDA is 16 mg per day for men and 14 mg per day for women. Foods containing significant amounts of niacin are liver, meat, poultry, fish, whole-grains and nuts.

**Vitamin $B_5$ (pantothenic acid)** is necessary for a variety of life-sustaining tasks such as generating energy from food, synthesizing essential fats, and the function of your adrenal glands.  Adequate intake of vitamin $B_5$ for adults is 5 mg per day. Good sources include organ meats, eggs, fish and shellfish, poultry, soybeans, beans, dairy foods, avocado, and mushrooms.

**Vitamin $B_6$ (pyridoxine)** is needed for protein and red-blood cell metabolism. Your body also requires vitamin $B_6$ to make hemoglobin.  For men and women up to 50 years old, the RDA is 1.3 mg per day.  After 50, the RDA increases to 1.7 mg per day for men and 1.5 mg for women.  Vitamin $B_6$ is found in a wide variety of foods including fortified cereals, beans, meat, poultry, fish, and some fruits and vegetables.

**Vitamin $B_7$ (biotin)** functions as a coenzyme in the synthesis of fat, glycogen and amino acids.  An adequate intake of biotin is 30 mcg per day. A varied diet should provide enough biotin for most people.  Liver, yeast and egg yokes are particularly rich food sources.  It is also found in smaller amounts in fruit, meat and cheese.

**Vitamin B₉ (folate or folic acid)** helps produce and maintain new cells which is particularly important during periods of rapid cell division and growth such as in infancy and during pregnancy.  Folate is needed to make DNA and RNA, the building blocks of cells. It is also thought to prevent DNA changes that may lead to cancer.  For most adults, the RDA of folate is 400 mcg per day.  Of course, woman who are expecting or nursing need more folate.  Cooked dry beans and peas, peanuts, oranges, dark-green-leafy vegetables and green peas are folate-rich foods.

**Vitamin B₁₂ (cyanocobalamin)** enables your body to manufacture healthy red-blood cells. It also assists in the transmission of electrical signals between nerve cells.  The recommended dietary allowance is 2.4 mcg per day.  Vitamin B₁₂ is found in fortified cereals, meat, fish and poultry.

**Calcium** is a mineral with several important functions.  Most of the calcium in your body is used to support the structure of your bones and teeth.  A small amount of calcium is in your blood, muscle, and the fluid between your cells.  Calcium is also needed for muscle contraction, blood vessel contraction and expansion, the secretion of hormones and enzymes, and sending messages through the nervous system.  For most adults, adequate intake is 1,000 mg per day.  Foods rich in calcium are milk, yogurt, natural cheeses (such as cheddar, Swiss and mozzarella), canned fish with soft bones such as salmon and sardines, and dark-green-leafy vegetables. Eight ounces of milk (whole or skim) contains 30 percent of your RDA.

**Chromium** is important in the metabolism of fats and carbohydrates and in controlling blood sugar levels.  It is an activator of several enzymes needed to drive numerous chemical reactions necessary to life.  For men and women up to 50 years old, an adequate intake of chromium is 35 and 25 mcg per day respectively.  After 50, the suggested adequate intake drops to 30 mcg per day for men and 20 for women.  Whole grains, ready-to-eat bran cereals, seafood, green beans, broccoli, prunes, nuts, peanut butter, and potatoes are rich in chromium.  One-half cup of chopped broccoli provides about 35 percent of your chromium RDA.

**Iodine** is a basic component of the thyroid hormone that regulates your metabolic rate.  Lack of iodine can cause a number of physical and mental abnormalities. RDA for adult men and women is 150 mcg per day.  Iodized salt, sea food and plants grown in iodine-rich soil are good sources of iodine. A three-ounce serving of cooked haddock contains about 125 mcg of iodine.

**Iron** is an important mineral that aids the transport of oxygen in your body and is also needed for the regulation of cell growth.  The RDA for iron is 8 mg per day for men and 18 mg per day for pre-menopausal women.

Foods rich in iron are shrimp, clams, mussels, oysters, sardines, lean meats (especially beef), organ meats, turkey (dark meat), spinach, cooked dry beans, peas, lentils, and whole-grain breads and cereals. Three ounces of beef liver has approximately 50 percent of your iron RDA, and fortified cereals can provide from 50 to 100 percent of your RDA.

| Mineral | Ages | | | |
|---|---|---|---|---|
| | 19-30 | 31-50 | 51-70 | 70+ |
| **Calcium** (mg) | 1000 | 1000 | 1200 | 1200 |
| **Chromium** (mcg) | 35 | 35 | 30 | 30 |
| **Copper** (mcg) | 900 | 900 | 900 | 900 |
| **Fluoride** (mg) | 4 | 4 | 4 | 4 |
| **Iodine** (mcg) | 150 | 150 | 150 | 150 |
| **Iron** (mg) | 8 | 8 | 8 | 8 |
| **Magnesium** (mg) | 400 | 420 | 420 | 420 |
| **Manganese** (mg) | 2.3 | 2.3 | 2.3 | 2.3 |
| **Molybdenum** (mcg) | 45 | 45 | 45 | 45 |
| **Phosphorus** (mg) | 700 | 700 | 700 | 700 |
| **Potassium** (mg) | 4700 | 4700 | 4700 | 4700 |
| **Selenium** (mcg) | 55 | 55 | 55 | 55 |
| **Zinc** (mg) | 11 | 11 | 11 | 11 |

**Table 7a: Mineral RDA for Men**

Values for calcium, chromium, fluoride & manganese are Adequate Intake. mcg = micrograms per day  mg = milligrams per day

| Mineral | Age | | | | | |
|---|---|---|---|---|---|---|
| | 19 to 30 | 31 to 50 | 51 to70 | 70+ | Preg | Lact |
| **Calcium** (mg) | 1000 | 1000 | 1200 | 1200 | 1000 | 1000 |
| **Chromium** (mcg) | 25 | 25 | 20 | 20 | 30 | 45 |
| **Copper** (mcg) | 900 | 900 | 900 | 900 | 1000 | 1300 |
| **Fluoride** (mg) | 3 | 3 | 3 | 3 | 3 | 3 |
| **Iodine** (mcg) | 150 | 150 | 150 | 150 | 220 | 290 |
| **Iron** (mg) | 18 | 18 | 8 | 8 | 27 | 9 |
| **Magnesium** (mg) | 310 | 320 | 320 | 320 | 355 | 315 |
| **Manganese** (mg) | 1.8 | 1.8 | 1.8 | 1.8 | 2.0 | 2.6 |
| **Molybdenum** (mcg) | 45 | 45 | 45 | 45 | 50 | 50 |
| **Phosphorus** (mg) | 700 | 700 | 700 | 700 | 700 | 700 |
| **Potassium** (mg) | 4700 | 4700 | 4700 | 4700 | 4700 | 5100 |
| **Selenium** (mcg) | 55 | 55 | 55 | 55 | 60 | 70 |
| **Zinc** (mg) | 8 | 8 | 8 | 8 | 8 | 8 |

**Table 7b: Mineral RDA for Women**

Preg = pregnant   Lact = lactating  mcg = micrograms per day  mg = milligrams per day. Calcium, chromium, fluoride & manganese values are Adequate Intake.

**Magnesium** is needed for hundreds of biochemical reactions in your body.  It helps maintain normal muscle and nerve function, keeps heart rhythm steady, supports a healthy immune system, and keeps bones strong. The RDA is 420 mg per day for men and 320 for women.  Dark-green-leafy vegetables, fish, some beans and peas, nuts and seeds, and whole grains are good sources of magnesium.  One-half cup of cooked spinach has 75 mg of magnesium.

**Phosphorus** in combination with calcium is necessary for the formation of bones and teeth.  Phosphorus is also involved in the metabolism of fats, carbohydrates and proteins, and in the effective utilization of many of the B vitamins.  The RDA for adults is 700 mg per day.  Rich sources of phosphorus are dairy products, meat, and fish. Phosphorus is also present in most soft drinks. Generally, a diet that provides adequate amounts of calcium and protein also provides a sufficient amount of phosphorus.

**Potassium** is involved in proper nerve function, muscle control and blood pressure regulation. (People engaged in vigorous exercise may need more potassium to replace that lost during exercise.) Low potassium levels can cause muscle cramping and cardiovascular irregularities. Adequate intake for men and women is 4,700 mg per day. Potassium-rich foods include baked white or sweet potatoes, cooked leafy greens, winter (orange) squash, bananas, oranges, dried fruits (such as apricots and prunes), and cooked dry beans and lentils. A medium-size baked potato contains about 600 mg of potassium.

**Selenium** is an essential trace element that assists enzymes involved in antioxidant protection and thyroid hormone metabolism. The RDA is 55 mcg per day for men and women. The most important sources in American diets are meats, fish and grains. Three ounces of cooked cod provide about 32 mcg of selenium.

**Zinc** is an essential mineral that stimulates the activity of approximately 100 enzymes that promote biochemical reactions in your body. Zinc supports a healthy immune system needed for wound healing, and helps maintain your sense of taste and smell. The RDA for zinc is 11 mg per day for men and 8 mg per day for women. Oysters contain more zinc per serving than any other food. Other good sources are red meat, poultry, beans, nuts, certain seafood, whole grains, dairy products and fortified breakfast cereals which can provide from 50 to 100 percent of your RDA.

## You Need Fiber

Fiber is an important part of a healthy diet. **You need to consume fiber to assist your digestive system**. According to the Harvard University School of Public Health, adequate fiber intake reduces the risk of developing various conditions, including heart disease, diabetes, diverticular disease, and constipation.

Three fibers that are eaten on a regular basis are cellulose, hemicellulose and pectin. Hemicellulose is found in the hulls of different grains like wheat; e.g., wheat bran is hemicellulose. Cellulose is the structural component of plants, and gives vegetables their familiar shape. Pectin is found most often in fruits, is soluble in water but non-digestible, and is usually referred to as "water-soluble fiber." The best fiber sources are:
- **Whole-grain** breads, whole-grain cereals, whole-wheat pasta and brown rice contain a great deal of hemicellulose fiber.
- **Fruits** are pectin rich (the water-soluble fiber). The skin on fruits are loaded with phytonutrients and fiber. So do not peal an apple. Eat it with the

skin on and get a fiber and nutrient boost.

- **Most berries** (such as bilberries, raspberries) have even more fiber than a comparable weight of most other fruit selections.
- **Vegetables** have lots of cellulose fiber.  Again the skin is particularly high in fiber.  When you eat a baked potato, eat it skin and all – everything – everything that is except the butter or sour cream.
- **Peas and beans** are high fiber foods that are also a complete protein when eaten with a whole grain food, or nuts, or seeds.
- **Nuts and seeds** add fiber to your diet.

When you eat fiber, in any of its forms, it simply passes straight through, untouched by but aiding your digestive system.  Zero calories absorbed!

**Adults should get a least 20 to 35 grams of dietary fiber per day**. How much fiber is in the foods you eat?  An apple has 3 grams of fiber, a tangerine has 2 grams, ½ cup cabbage contains 2 grams, a tomato has 2 grams, ½ cup broccoli has 1 gram, ½ cup of lima beans contains 4 grams, 1 cup of brown rice has 3 grams, 1 cup of whole-wheat cereal holds 3 grams and 1 slice of whole-wheat bread contains 2 grams of fiber.

## Drink Lots of Water

The average adult female body is about 52 percent water, while the average adult male is approximately 63 percent water.  If you are average, everyday you lose about 10 cups of water when you breathe, perspire, and excrete waste. Because water is needed for almost every biochemical and physiologic process in your body, to maintain your body's water balance you must replace this lost water.  (The water in your body is said to be balanced, when your water intake from all sources equals your loss of water.)

Typically, the food you eat every day contains about 3 cups of mostly concealed water. When you metabolize the food you eat, you create another cup of water.  That leaves about six cups that must be replaced by the liquids you drink – even more when you exercise.  It appears, therefore, that the long-established wisdom advocating that you drink eight glasses of water per day (or any other healthy beverage such as tea or fruit juice) is not far from the mark.

## Use Salt Sparingly

Sodium and sodium chloride (salt) normally occur in small quantities in many natural foods. Salt and sodium-containing ingredients are also frequently found in high amounts in processed foods, such as canned soup and baked goods.  People also add salt during food preparation and to the food they eat.  Although sodium plays an important role in your body, many studies have demonstrated that high sodium intake is also associated with high blood pressure.  In your body, sodium retains water expanding blood volume which in turn raises blood pressure.  Moreover, although some questions remain, evidence suggests that many adults who are predisposed to high blood pressure (for example having a parent who has high blood pressure) can reduce their chances of developing high blood pressure by consuming less sodium.

Most Americans consume too much sodium.  The U.S. Department of Health and Human Services and the Department of Agriculture Dietary Guidelines recommend that healthy adults **limit sodium intake to 2,400 mg per day.**  (Note that one level teaspoon of salt contains about 2,300 mg of sodium.)  Individuals who have high blood pressure and are also salt sensitive are frequently advised to limit their sodium intake even further.

## Not Too Much Sugar

Sugars are carbohydrates that come in many forms.  Sugar is found naturally in fruits, some vegetables, milk, breads, cereals and grains, and is often added to foods during processing, preparation and when eating.  Added sugar and naturally occurring sugars are chemically identical and your body cannot distinguish between them.  Cake, cookies, candy and many soft drinks contain large amounts of added sugar that supply a large number of "nutritionally-empty calories."  Only very active people with high calorie needs can afford to consume any quantity of these sugar-laden foods.  **Sugar should be used sparingly** by people with low calorie needs and in moderation by most other healthy adults.  (Contrary to what many believe, the latest scientific evidence seems to indicate diets high in sugar do not cause diabetes.  Rather, scientific evidence indicates that adult-onset diabetes occurs most often in those who are overweight.)

## Phytonutrients

Phytonutrients are not vitamins or minerals.  Rather they are the beneficial compounds that give fruits and vegetables their many colors. "Phyto" comes from the Greek word for "plant," and that is where phytonutrients are found – in plant foods such as fruits, vegetables, whole grains, dried beans, nuts and seeds.  Unlike traditional macronutrients and micronutrients (protein, fat, vitamins and minerals), phytonutrients are not necessary for life; i.e., they are not required for normal metabolism and their absence will not result in a deficiency disease.  Despite this, research is expanding as evidence grows that phytonutrients have many beneficial qualities such as assisting the function of the immune system, reducing inflammation, acting directly against viruses, and playing a crucial role in preventing or reducing the risk of a number of chronic ailments, including heart disease, diabetes and cancer.

**One of the most important roles of phytonutrients is as an antioxidant.** Free radicals, which are by-products of energy metabolism, can damage cells and are thought to contribute to the development of cardiovascular disease and cancer. When antioxidant molecules encounter free radicals they neutralize them – limiting the damage. Your body needs more antioxidants as you grow older, because your body's ability to repair itself diminishes as you age. Antioxidants are also thought to help prevent cell damage by environmental carcinogens.

Scientists understanding of phytonutrients is still in its infancy. Despite this, about one thousand phytonutrients have been identified to date and with ever expanding research new compounds are continually being discovered and organized into classes. The best known phytonutrient classes are carotenoids and polyphenols.

**Carotenoids** are contained in the yellow, orange, and red pigment in fruits and vegetables, as well as in dark-green-leafy vegetables (where the usual yellow color is masked by the vegetable's green pigment).

Some of the phytonutrients within the carotenoids class are alpha-carotene (contained in carrots); beta-carotene (in broccoli, sweet potato, pumpkin and carrots); beta-cryptoxanthin (in citrus fruits, peaches and apricots); lutein (in leafy greens such as kale, spinach and turnip greens); lycopene (in tomatoes, tomato paste, guava, pink grapefruit and watermelon); and zeaxanthin (in green vegetables and citrus fruit).

**Polyphenol** compounds are natural components of a wide variety of plants. Foods rich in polyphenols include apples, red wine, red grapes, grape juice, strawberries, raspberries, blueberries, cranberries, onions, tea, and certain nuts. Polyphenols are further subdivided into  flavonoids and nonflavonoids.

Some phytonutrients in the flavonoids subgroup are anthocyanins (in fruits); catechins (found in tea and red wine); flavanones (in citrus fruit) flavones (in most fruits and vegetables); flavonols (in most fruits, vegetables, tea and red wine); and isoflavones (in soybeans). The nonflavonoids subgroup contains ellagic acid (found in strawberries, blueberries and raspberries).

# 4. NUTRITION FOR HEALTH

## Guidelines for Healthy Eating

No single food can supply all the nutrients you need in the amounts you need. The most important factors in nutrition are variety, variety, variety!  **Variety is the key to a nutritious diet**.  As a means of setting strategies for food selection, the U.S. Department of Health and Human Services and the Department of Agriculture issue Dietary Guidelines every five years.  In 2015 MyPyramid was replaced with **MyPlate** (see figure below).  The 2015 Dietary Guidelines recommend the following:

• **Make Half your Plate Fruits and Vegetables:** Eat red, orange, and dark-green vegetables, such as tomatoes, sweet potatoes, and broccoli.  Eat fruit, vegetables, or unsalted nuts as snacks.

• **Switch to Skim or 1% Milk:** Both have the same amount of calcium and other essential nutrients as whole milk, but less fat and calories.  If lactose intolerant, try calcium-fortified soy products as an alternative to dairy foods.

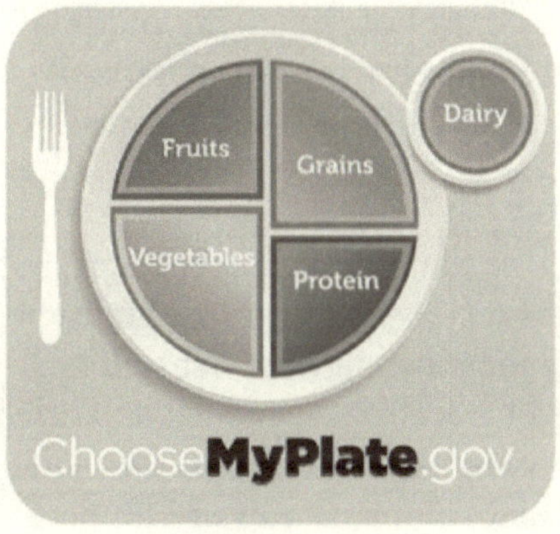


• **Make at least Half your Grains Whole:** Choose 100% wholegrain cereals, breads, crackers, rice, and pasta.  Check the ingredients list on food packages to find whole-grain foods.

• **Vary your Protein Food choices:** Twice a week, make seafood the protein on your plate.  Eat beans, a natural source of fiber and protein.  Keep meat and poultry portions small & lean.

• **Choose Foods and Drinks with little or No Added Sugars:** Drink water instead of sugary drinks. Select fruit for dessert.  Eat sugary desserts less often.  Choose 100% fruit juice instead of fruit-flavored drinks.

• **Look Out for Salt (sodium) in Foods you Buy:** Compare sodium in foods like soup, bread, and frozen meals and choose the foods with lower numbers. Add spices or herbs to season food without adding salt.

• **Eat Fewer Foods that are High in Solid Fats:** Make major sources of saturated fats – such as cakes, cookies, ice cream, pizza, cheese, sausages, and hot dogs – occasional choices, not everyday foods.  Select lean cuts of meats or poultry and fat-free or low-fat milk, yogurt, and cheese.  Switch from solid fats to oils when preparing food.

• **To Maintain a Healthy Weight:** Basically enjoy your food, but eat less. Stay within your personal calorie limit. (Note that caloric needs are not covered here.  See *Weight Control - U.S. Edition* by Vincent Antonetti, PhD, for example.)  Think before you eat:  Is it worth the calories? Avoid oversized portions.  Use a smaller plate, bowl, and glass.  Stop eating when you are satisfied, not full.

• **Know your personal Daily Calorie Limit:** Keep that calorie number in mind when deciding what to eat.  ( Again, see *Weight Control - U.S. Edition* by Vincent Antonetti, PhD.)  Use a food log to keep track of how much you eat.

• **When Eating out Check posted Calorie Amounts:** Choose lower calorie menu options.  Select dishes that include vegetables, fruits, and/or whole grains.  Order a smaller portion or share when eating out.  Cook more often at home, where you are in control of what's in your food.

• **If you Drink Alcoholic beverages, do so Sensibly:** Limit should be 1 drink a day for women or to 2 drinks a day for men.

## Basic Food Groups

In this section we describe the various food groups, indicate what constitutes a serving size, and focus on the best foods within each group.  (The foods in **bold font** are generally the most nutrient-dense foods – the best of the best.)

**Fruit Group**:  Includes fresh, frozen, canned and dried fruits and fruit juices. Usually, a serving is 1 cup.  A serving from the fruit group consists of 1 cup of fresh, frozen or canned fruit, or 1 cup of 100 percent fruit juice, or ½ cup of dried fruit.  This group can be divided further into citrus fruits, berries and grapes, and other fruits.

**Citrus fruits**: There are many excellent citrus choices including **oranges, grapefruit, lemons, limes, kiwifruit and kumquats**.  All are low calorie foods that contain a negligible amount of  fat and cholesterol, are high in vitamin C, and most have significant amounts of vitamin A, potassium and dietary fiber.

**Berries & grapes**: Among the fruits in this grouping are **blackberries, blueberries, raspberries, strawberries, cranberries, gooseberries, purple grapes, black currents, raisins, and cherries**.  Every fresh berry and grape is low calorie, with no fat or cholesterol, and all have small amounts of multiple micronutrients and a fair amount of dietary fiber. (Strawberries are also rich in vitamin C.)  Some researchers claim that the blue and black-colored berries are packed with more disease-fighting antioxidants than any other fruit or vegetable. Of course, dark-red and purple grape contain the phytonutrient flavonol, the same antioxidant believed to give red wine its heart-protecting benefits.

**Other fruits**: This large subgroup includes a number of healthy foods such as **apples, apricots, bananas, cantaloupe, figs, mangos, papayas, peaches, pears, pineapples, plums, prunes and watermelon**. Again, most are low calorie, contain no fat or cholesterol, and are loaded with vitamins, minerals and phytonutrients. In addition, apples, apricots, figs, peaches, pears, pineapples, plums, prunes are good sources of dietary fiber. Cantaloupe is also high in vitamin C and watermelon contains the phytonutrient lycopene.

**Vegetable Group**: Includes fresh, frozen, dried and canned vegetables and vegetable juices. In general, 1 cup from the vegetable group consists of 1 cup of raw or cooked vegetables or vegetable juice, or 2 cups of raw-leafy greens. This group can be broken down further into dark-green-leafy vegetables, orange-colored vegetables, starchy vegetables and other vegetables.

**Dark-green-leafy vegetables**: Every food in this category (which includes **bok choy, collard greens, kale, mustard greens, romaine lettuce, spinach, Swiss chard and turnip greens**) is low calorie with no fat or cholesterol, and is packed with micronutrients, especially vitamins A and C, calcium, iron, potassium and folate, as well as dietary fiber.

**Orange-colored vegetables**: The best in this subgroup are **carrots, orange-bell peppers, pumpkin, sweet potatoes, yams and winter squash**. All have negligible fat and cholesterol and are high in vitamin A, potassium and dietary fiber.

**Starchy vegetables**: This grouping overlaps somewhat with the orange-colored vegetable subgroup and the grains group. Among the foods included are **white potatoes, sweet potatoes, yams, yellow corn, and brown rice**. These vegetables are generally high in complex carbohydrates, B vitamins, potassium and dietary fiber.

**Other vegetables**: This extensive category contains **asparagus, broccoli, Brussels sprouts, cabbage, cauliflower, celery, cucumber, fennel, green beans, parsley, and summer squash**. The preceding are low calorie foods that contain a negligible amount of fat and cholesterol, and most have significant amounts of vitamins A and C, potassium, calcium, iron, other micronutrients and dietary fiber. Also in this category are **eggplant, garlic, leeks, onions and mushrooms** which contain few calories, no cholesterol, and important amounts of potassium, calcium, iron and other micronutrients, as well as dietary fiber. **Red peppers and tomatoes** are low-calorie vegetables with no cholesterol that are loaded with vitamins A and C, iron and dietary fiber. Tomatoes also contain the phytonutrient lycopene. **Avocado and olives** contain some beneficial monounsaturated and polyunsaturated fat, but no cholesterol.  Avocados are relatively high in potassium and vitamin A, while olives have significant amounts of iron and calcium.

: Includes all foods made from wheat, rice, oats, cornmeal and barley, such as bread, pasta, oatmeal, breakfast cereals and grits.  Generally, 1 ounce from the grains group consists of 1 thin slice of bread, or 1 cup of ready-to-eat cereal, or ½ cup of cooked rice, pasta or cooked cereal.  <u>At least half of the grains eaten should be whole grains</u>.

Grains are the seeds of  varied grasses grown for food.  The outermost layer of the grain is an inedible husk, called chaff.  The next layer is the bran, a protective coating rich in fiber.  When this layer is removed, the product is described as pearled or polished.  Inside the bran is the endosperm (the starchy part of a grain) and the germ, the part highest in nutrients (e.g., wheat germ).  Whole grains have all these components intact.  Refined grains have the husk, bran, and germ removed.  Many foods are a mixture of whole and refined grains.  Check the ingredient list for the words "whole grain" or "whole wheat" to determine if a food is made from a whole grain.  In the United States, to be labeled "whole grain" a food must contain more than 51 percent whole grain by weight.

 include: **barley, buckwheat, bulgur, corn, millet, oats, brown rice, rye, wheat and wild rice**.  Some whole-grain foods are: **whole-wheat bread, whole-grain ready-to-eat cereal, whole-wheat crackers, oatmeal, popcorn, whole-wheat pasta**, and whole barley (in beef-barley soup).  All grains are low in fat and contain no cholesterol.  Whole grains are good sources of complex carbohydrates and dietary fiber, as well as several B vitamins (thiamin, riboflavin, niacin, and folate), vitamin E, and minerals (iron, magnesium, and selenium).

: Generally, 1 ounce equivalent from this group consists of 1 ounce of lean meat, poultry, or fish, or 1 egg, or 1 tablespoon of peanut butter, or ¼ cup cooked dry beans, or ½ cup of nuts or seeds.  This group can be divided further into subgroups consisting of meat and foul, fish, eggs, beans, and nuts and seeds.

:  **Skinless white-meat chicken and turkey** are relatively low calorie, low fat, low cholesterol foods that are powerful sources of high-quality protein, vitamin $B_6$, riboflavin, niacin, phosphorus and potassium.  Most meats, even **lean meats**, are higher in fat and calories than chicken and turkey, but meats do provide high-quality protein and some important nutrients such as iron and B-vitamins.

: Most fish are good choices including **cod, halibut, herring, mackerel, salmon, sardines, scallops, shrimp, snapper, trout and tuna.**  Nearly all fish contain high levels of essential-fatty acids.  (Oily cold-water fish such as wild salmon, sardines, herring, mackerel and tuna are high in omega-3 essential-fatty acid. Trout also has comparatively high omega-3 content.)

All fish are relatively low-calorie foods and are good sources of the fat-soluble vitamins A and D. (Fish-liver oils have high levels of fat soluble vitamins, and have been used as dietary supplements for many years.) Nutritionally, seafood is better known for its dietary minerals than for its vitamins. This is because some minerals in fish, such as iodine and selenium, are not available at the same levels in most other non-marine foods. Fish are also a good source of iron and potassium.

There is, however, a downside to eating fish. Some fish are contaminated with mercury, PCBs, dioxins and other environmental pollutants. Mercury is a toxic heavy metal that can accumulate in certain fish species. Large predatory fish such as shark, swordfish, king mackerel and tilefish have the highest concentration of mercury and other environmental contaminates. Canned white albacore tuna, a commonly eaten fish, contains higher levels of mercury than canned light tuna . The U.S. Food and Drug Administration advises adults to eat no more than six ounces of high-mercury fish per week.

PCBs are potential human carcinogens that find their way into fresh waters and oceans where they are absorbed by fish. A recent study reported that PCB levels in farmed salmon, especially those in from Europe, were about seven times higher than in wild salmon.

For further information about the safety of fish you catch locally, have your client visit the U.S. Environmental Protection Agency's Fish Advisory website: www.epa.gov/ost/fish or contact your state or local health department. If no advice is available, eat no more than six ounces per week of fish caught from local waters and do not consume any other fish that week.

According to the University of Michigan Integrative Medicine Department, pregnant and nursing women, and young children, should avoid shark, swordfish, king mackerel and tilefish, and strictly limit the amount of other contaminated fish consumed.

**Eggs:** Current dietary guidelines and the latest research concerning egg consumption appear to be at odds. On the one hand, because a typical egg yoke contains saturated fat and 300 mg of cholesterol, the latest dietary guidelines recommend that egg yolks and whole eggs be used in moderation (up to one egg per day), but that egg whites and egg substitutes can be used freely since they contain no cholesterol and little or no fat.

On the other hand, others argue that if judged as a whole food and not simply as a source of cholesterol, positives such as the fact that eggs are low calorie, are loaded with high-quality protein, are a good source of vitamin E, etc, are apparent.  Moreover, researchers at the Harvard Medical School studied egg consumption among 120,000 nurses and other health professionals with normal cholesterol levels and reported no link between eating eggs and heart disease or stroke.

Some medical researchers advise that, if one is at low risk (i.e., does not smoke, exercises regularly, eats a healthy diet and has no family history of heart disease or stroke) and chooses to begin eating eggs, they should have a blood test four to six weeks after they start eating eggs to determine the impact on their total and LDL cholesterol.  Based on the test results, your client and her doctor can decide – yes or no to her eating more eggs.

**Beans:**  Among the foods in this important subgroup are **black beans, cannelloni beans, dried peas, fava beans, garbanzo beans, red kidney beans, lentils, lima beans, navy beans, and pinto beans**.  All beans are inexpensive, low-fat, plant-protein-rich foods that are good sources of B vitamins, potassium, iron, dietary fiber and isoflavones (important phytonutrients).

**Nuts and Seeds:** This category consists of **almonds, cashews, hazelnuts, peanuts, pecans, pistachio nuts, walnuts, flaxseed, pumpkin seeds, sesame seeds, sunflower seeds**, and others.  Because nuts and seeds contain significant amounts of essential-fatty acids, they are comparatively high-calorie foods.  Most nuts and seeds have a good amount of dietary fiber, vitamin E, potassium, iron and folate.  Almonds, cashews, peanuts, and pine nuts contain a significant quantity of plant protein and essential-fatty acids.  Walnuts, flaxseed and pumpkin seeds are important sources of plant-based omega-3 fatty acids.

**Soy:** The soybean is the most widely grown legume.  Healthful soy foods such as **tofu, soy nuts, soymilk, soybean oil, and soy protein** are made from soybeans.  All contain a significant amount of plant-based <u>complete protein</u> and omega-3 fatty acid as well as vitamin E, potassium, iron and folate.  Soy nuts are also high in dietary fiber.

Soybeans, tofu, and other soy-based foods are an excellent alternative to red meat.  But there  are some suspected dangers from too much soy.  So advise your client not to overdo it.  The Harvard University School of Public Health recommends two to four servings of soy foods per week as a good goal.  Furthermore, they caution adults not to take supplements that contain concentrated soy protein or soy extracts, such as isoflavones.

**Milk Group:** Includes liquid milk and all products and foods made from milk such yogurt and cheese.  (Foods that have little or no calcium such as cream, butter and cream cheese are not in this group.)  In general, 1 cup from the milk group consists of 1 cup of milk or yogurt, or 1½ ounces of natural cheese, or 2 ounces of processed cheese.

**Milk, yogurt and natural cheeses** are high in calcium and protein. **Milk** is also often fortified with vitamin D.  In addition to calcium and protein, **yogurt** is a particularly wholesome food providing live active bacteria cultures which promote gastrointestinal health.  Most choices in this group should be fat free or low fat.

**Oils Group:** Includes vegetable oils and foods such as **nuts, olives, oily fish, avocados**, mayonnaise, soft margarine and some salad dressings.  You should limit the intake of saturated fats – that is any fat of animal origin.

The oils group overlaps somewhat with many of the others.  Liquid oils, however, are unique to this group.  **Corn oil, flaxseed oil,  safflower oil, sesame oil, soybean oil and sunflower oil** are polyunsaturated; whereas, **canola oil, olive oil and peanut oil** are monounsaturated.  All these oils are high in calories and essential-fatty acids.  Essential-fatty acids promote absorption of the fat-soluble vitamins A, D, E, and K. Flaxseed, canola and soybean oil contain omega-3 fatty acids.  (Note, when purchasing olive oil, choose an oil that is labeled "extra-virgin" or "virgin."  Virgin olive oils are produced from the first pressing of the olives,  are unrefined and as a result are more healthful.)

## Vitamin & Mineral Supplements

Even though most adults can get all the vitamins and minerals they need by merely consuming a variety of nutritious foods (from the fruit group, the vegetable group, the grains group, the meat and beans group, the milk group, and the oils group), **many physicians recommend a daily multi-vitamin/mineral supplement as a kind of insurance policy**.

Be aware that some micronutrients, such as the fat-soluble vitamin A, can be harmful if taken in large quantities.  To be safe your multi-vitamin/mineral supplement should contain no more than 100 percent of the recommended dietary allowance (RDA) for each vitamin or mineral. Generally, you don't need the high doses in multi-vitamin/mineral supplements labeled "therapeutic" or "extra-strength."  There may be medical reasons for taking larger amounts of a vitamin or mineral than the RDA provides, but check with your doctor first.  For example, a physician may advise a pregnant woman to take an iron supplement, and women who could become pregnant to take folic acid in addition to consuming folate-rich foods to reduce the risk of some serious birth defects.  Adults over age 50 and vegetarians who do not eat animal foods may be advised to get their vitamin $B_{12}$ from a supplement or from fortified foods. People with little exposure to sunlight may need a vitamin D supplement, and individuals who seldom eat dairy products or other rich sources of calcium may need to take a calcium supplement.

Dietary supplement choices include not only vitamins and minerals, but also herbal products and many other widely available substances. Herbal products, however, usually provide only small amounts of vitamins and minerals and their health value is currently being studied.

## For Senior Citizens

As you age, adequate protein intake and body protein reserves are more important than ever, especially during times of emotional and physical stress. Body proteins are constantly being made and used during your lifetime to maintain the functions of the cells and organs, and protein is needed to help to prevent muscle loss. As already mentioned, good sources of protein-rich foods are meats, fish, eggs, dairy products, dried beans and peas, and soy products.

**Vitamin $B_{12}$ can be a problem nutrient for older adults.** Vitamin $B_{12}$ enables your body to manufacture healthy red-blood cells and assists in the transmission of electrical signals between nerve cells. The acid in your stomach helps release vitamin $B_{12}$ from the protein in the food you eat. This must occur before vitamin $B_{12}$ is absorbed in your intestines. But as you age, the amount of stomach acid you produce decreases. Less hydrochloric acid lessens the amount of vitamin $B_{12}$ separated from proteins in foods and can result in poor absorption of vitamin $B_{12}$. Vitamin $B_{12}$ is found naturally in meat, fish, poultry, eggs and fortified cereals. Recent studies have revealed that up to 30 percent of adults aged 50 years and older may also have atrophic gastritis, an increased growth of intestinal bacteria, that renders them unable to normally absorb vitamin $B_{12}$ in food. They are, however, able to absorb the synthetic vitamin $B_{12}$ added to fortified foods and dietary supplements. As a result, fortified foods and vitamin supplements may be the best sources of vitamin $B_{12}$ for adults 50 years and older. In fact the newest U.S. Modified Food Guide Pyramid for 70 plus Adults recommends that this age group take a dietary supplement for vitamin $B_{12}$, calcium and vitamin D. (Vitamin D supplements are particularly important for older adults with limited exposure to sunlight.)

## Organic Food – Yes or No?

Buying organic fruits, vegetables, dairy, meat and poultry can cost as much as 50 to 100 percent more than conventional non-organic foods. Is organic worth the extra cost? Read on.

"Organic" refers to the methods farmers grow and process agricultural products, including fruits, vegetables, grains, dairy products and meat. Farmers who grow organic produce and meat don't use conventional methods to fertilize, control weeds or prevent livestock disease. As an example, rather than using chemical weed killers, organic farmers conduct sophisticated crop rotations and mulch to keep weeds at bay. Instead of synthetic pesticides organic farms use helpful insects and birds, mating disruption or traps to reduce pests and disease. In place of chemical fertilizers, organic farms employ natural fertilizers, such as manure or compost. Animals on organic farms eat organically grown feed, aren't confined 100 percent of the time and are raised without antibiotics or synthetic growth hormones.

## Organic Food Labeling

The U.S. Department of Agriculture has established an organic certification program that requires all organic foods to meet strict government standards. These standards regulate how such foods are grown, handled and processed. Any farmer or food manufacturer who labels and sells a product as organic must be USDA certified as meeting the following standards.

**100 percent Organic:** Only products that are completely organic or with all organic ingredients can be labeled 100 percent organic and can be affixed with a USDA seal.

**Organic:** Products that are at least 95 percent organic can also carry a USDA seal.

**Made with Organic Ingredients:** These are products that contain at least 70 percent organic ingredients. The organic seal can not be used on these packages.

Foods containing less than 70 percent organic ingredients cannot use the organic seal or the word "organic" on their product label. Package labeling standards are summarized in Table 7.

| Package Label | Contents | USDA Organic Label |
|---|---|---|
| 100 percent Organic | 100% organic | Can use USDA Organic Label |
| Organic | At least 95% organic | Can use USDA Organic Label |
| Organic Ingredients | At least 70% organic | Label can not be used |

**Table 8: USDA Organic Labeling Standards**

## Is Organic Worth the Cost?

Most organic food costs more than non-organic conventional food products. Higher prices are due to more expensive farming practices, tighter government regulations and lower crop yields. The question is are organic foods worth the extra cost? Critics argue that we're wasting our money because there's no proof that conventionally produced foods pose significant health risks.

Some studies have linked chemical weed killers, synthetic pesticides and synthetic growth hormones in non-organic food to everything from headaches to cancer to birth defects. This growing body of research shows that pesticides and other contaminants are more prevalent in the foods we eat, in our bodies, and in the environment than we thought – but quite a few experts maintain that the levels of these alien substances in non-organic foods are safe for most healthy adults. Some scientists are also worried about the antibiotics given to most farm animals. Many are the same antibiotics we humans rely on, and overuse of these drugs has already enabled bacteria to develop resistance to them, rendering them less effective in combating infection in humans.

Although the USDA certifies organic food, it doesn't claim that organic products are safer or more nutritious. Indeed, there is no conclusive evidence that shows that organic food is more nutritious than conventionally grown non-organic food.

In this writer's opinion, if you can afford it, buy local and organic but you don't have to buy organic across the board because not all organic-labeled products offer added health value. For example, it's worth paying more for the "dirty dozen": peaches, strawberries, nectarines, apples, spinach, celery, pears, sweet bell peppers, cherries, potatoes, lettuce, and imported grapes. These fragile fruits and vegetables often require more pesticides to fight off bugs compared to hardier produce, such as asparagus and broccoli. But you can also pass on organic seafood and shampoo, which have labels that are often misleading.

You can also find organic food at most farmer's markets, and many of the farmers don't charge an organic premium. For listings of local farmer's markets, go to http://www.ams.usda.gov/farmersmarkets. Another alternative is to buy a share in a community-supported organic farm. You'll get a weekly supply of produce from spring until fall. Costs are reasonable although most farms will require you to work a few hours a month distributing or picking produce. The cost savings can be substantial. Go to http://www.sare.org for a list of community-supported farms.

## Is Vegetarianism for You?

A strict vegetarian diet is one that rejects all animal-based foods (including poultry, game, fish, shellfish or crustacean) and slaughter by-products. There are several variants of the diet. A generic term for both vegetarianism, veganism, and similar diets, is "plant-based" diets. The reasons for choosing a plant-based diet are varied and may be centered on morality, religion, culture, ethics, aesthetics, environment, society, economy, politics, taste, nutrition or health.

## Types of Vegetarians

When deciding what type of vegetarian you might want to be, think about what foods you want to include or avoid. Understanding the following popular vegetarian types may help you decide.

**1. Lacto-Ovo Vegetarians** do not eat animal flesh of any kind (including beef, pork, poultry, fish and shellfish) but they do eat eggs and dairy products. Some ovo-lacto vegetarians eat meat by-products (e.g. fats, bonemeal, gelatin) and use animal-derived products (leather etc.). This is the most practiced type of vegetarianism.

**2. Lacto-Vegetarians** do not eat animal flesh of any kind (including beef, pork, poultry, fish and shellfish) and do not eat meat or eggs – but do eat dairy products.

**3. Ovo-Vegetarians** do not eat animal flesh of any kind (including beef, pork, poultry, fish and shellfish) and do not eat meat or dairy products – but do eat eggs.

**4. Semi-Vegetarians** abstain from eating all meat and animal flesh with the exception of fish – although factory-farmed fish are usually avoided.. People are adopting this kind of diet, usually for health reasons or as a stepping stone to a fully vegetarian diet.

**5. Vegans** are strict vegetarians who do not eat meat of any kind and also do not eat eggs, dairy products, or processed foods containing these or other animal-derived ingredients. Many vegans also refrain from eating foods that are made using animal products even though the food may not contain animal products in the finished product, such as sugar and some wines.

## Becoming a Vegetarian

There are no set rules. The best way to move away from meat and become a vegetarian is to do it gradually. Becoming a vegetarian can be a process, not necessarily an overnight event. Some vegetarians would say that vegetarianism is more of a way of life, not simply what you put on your plate. If you're trying to determine what your first step to vegetarianism should be, these quick tips should help you make the transition.

    1. Read, talk and learn as much as you can about vegetarian health and diet. Knowledge is power! If you know any other vegetarians or vegans, ask them for tips or advice.

    2. Browse your local bookstore and buy a good vegetarian cookbook. Look for one that has a variety of recipes that are simple enough for everyday use.

**3**. Transform dishes that you already know and enjoy. For example, omit meatballs from your favorite spaghetti recipe, or replace them with a vegetarian substitute. Chances are, much of what you already eat could easily be made vegetarian.

**4**. Explore new foods. One technique is to try one new product every time you go food shopping. Most supermarkets carry non-dairy milks, meat alternatives, vegan frozen dinners, beside their standard selections of veggies, fruits, grains, beans, and nuts. In recent years, the many have a health food section which features vegan chips, dips, power bars, cereals, egg-free mayonnaise and even non-dairy cream cheese and ice cream. And try browsing in your local health food stores to see what new foods you can find.

**5**. Try it twice. If you disliked a particular food the first time, such as veggie burgers. Try them again later. Buy a different brand or prepare the burgers differently or with different seasonings and spices.

**6**. Try new restaurants: Chinese, Indian, Middle Eastern and Thai restaurants. Taste the many dishes and foods they have to offer.

## Vegetarian Nutrition

Properly planned vegetarian diets have been found to satisfy nutritional needs for all stages of life. Large-scale studies have shown vegetarian diets significantly lower the risk of colon cancer, heart disease, high blood pressure and other diseases. In fact, many health-care professionals think that <u>eating a healthy vegetarian diet</u> is one of the best things you can do for your short-term and long-term health.

Be sure to replace meat with healthy foods and eat a balanced diet. Vegetarian, vegan or not, you need to consider the health effects of what you eat. While eating an adequate amount of protein is important for vegetarians, getting sufficient calcium and iron (and if you're vegan vitamin $B_{12}$) are equally important

You must eat a variety of whole grains, vegetables and proteins, such as tofu or veggie burgers to stay full and healthy. A well-balanced vegetarian diet with plenty of whole grains, fruits and vegetables is one of the healthiest diets on the planet. You do, however, need to make sure you get ample amounts of the following vital nutrients and micronutrients.

**Protein:** Most people get too much protein – not too little of it. Women need about 45 grams a day and men need around 55 grams. One cup of tofu contains about 20 grams of protein. Lots of foods contain protein and if vegetarians eat a well-balanced diet, they are  undoubtedly consuming more than enough protein without even thinking about it. Lacto-ovo vegetarians get sufficient protein from eggs and dairy. Some high protein vegan foods include: tofu, veggie burgers, soy, lentils, chickpeas, nuts and seeds, brown rice and whole grains.

**Calcium:** Adults need calcium and smokers need even more calcium, as a smoker's absorption and retention levels are lower. Strong bones throughout life come from both calcium in the diet and exercise, so for optimum health, be sure to get both. Dairy products are a good source of calcium. Other calcium-rich foods are: spinach, collard greens, kale, soy milk, fortified orange juice, sesame seeds, broccoli, almonds, carrots, and rice milk.

**Iron:** Studies have found that iron levels in vegetarians and vegans, on average, were higher than those of the general population, showing that it's possible to get more than enough iron on a vegan diet. Again, to get enough iron eat a balanced diet including foods like tofu, lentils, spinach, soy, chickpeas and hummus.

**Vitamin $B_{12}$:** Vegetarians should not have to worry about vitamin $B_{12}$. $B_{12}$ deficiency is rare among vegans, vegetarians and non-vegetarians alike, but is a serious issue when it does occur. (Nutritional yeast is great source of vitamin $B_{12}$ and an incredibly tasty addition to just about everything, although miso and some seaweeds contain a small amount of $B_{12}$ as well.) Seniors are usually advised to get their vitamin $B_{12}$ from a supplement or from fortified foods.

## Vegan Nutrition

Nutritional guidelines for vegans are essentially similar to those for vegetarians, although being more restricted than the more popular lacto-ovo vegetarian diets, vegan eating plans need to ensure adequate intake of the nutrients and micronutrients listed below, by consuming the cited plant-food sources.

**Vitamin $B_2$ (Riboflavin):** Some studies have found vegans have a low intake of vitamin B2. Good sources of vitamin B2 are: whole grains, mushrooms, almonds, leafy green vegetables and yeast extracts.

**Vitamin $B_{12}$:** This micronutrient is absent from plant-foods, being found mainly in meat products, dairy products and eggs. Fortunately, vegans can obtain $B_{12}$ from a wide range of $B_{12}$-fortified foods. $B_{12}$-fortified foods include: yeast extracts, veggie-burger mixes, breakfast cereals, vegetable margarines and soy milk. Additionally, to be safe, vegans are often advised to take a $B_{12}$ supplement at least once a week.

**Vitamin D:** This critical vitamin is found in oily fish, eggs and dairy products. It is not found in plant foods. As with vitamin $B_{12}$, vegans can obtain vitamin D from vegetable margarines, soy milk and certain other foods that are fortified with vitamin D. Of course, vitamin D is also obtainable from sunshine.  Vegans who are confined indoors may be prescribed a vitamin D supplement.

**Iodine:**  Various studies have indicated some vegans have a low iodine intake.  Plant sources of iodine include: seaweeds, vegetables and grains, although the amount of iodine in vegetables and grains depends on the iodine content of the soil.

**Adequate Calorie Intake:**  Many plant-foods in a vegan diet are high in bulk and may satisfy hunger without providing sufficient calories.  Vegans should therefore watch their weight and calorie-intake to ensure they have adequate energy levels.

**Foods a Vegan** should keep on hand:  Soy milk (fortified with vitamin B12, vitamin D and calcium), fortified yeast extract, fortified breakfast cereals and dried seaweeds

## Become a Calorie Expert

Today, most food packages in the United States are required to list certain nutritional information.  The food labels on containers consist of several parts, including information on the front panel, and Nutrition Facts – usually on a side or rear panel.

The **Front Panel** often indicates if nutrients have been added – a case in point, "iodized salt" lets you know iodine has been added, and "enriched pasta" (or "enriched" grain of any type) means that thiamin, riboflavin, niacin, iron, and folic acid have been added.  The **Nutrition Facts label** (such as that on the side of a cereal box) indicates the number of calories and nutrients in a serving.  You can also use the label to compare similar foods. For instance, to determine which brand of a frozen dinner is lower in saturated fat, or which breakfast cereal contains more folic acid.  Look at the "% Daily Value" column to determine if a food is high or low in a particular nutrient.  The ingredient list on the Nutrition Facts label also discloses what is in the food, including any nutrients, fats, or sugars that have been added. Ingredients are in descending order by weight; i.e., the most abundant ingredient is listed first.

The Nutrition Facts label on food packages makes it possible to calculate the number of calories in a serving if you know that there are:

|  | Calories per gram | Calories per ounce |
|---|---|---|
| **Carbohydrates** | 4 | 110 |
| **Protein** | 4 | 110 |
| **Alcohol** | 7 | 200 |
| **Fat** | 9 | 260 |

<u>**Example**</u>  Determine the calories in a cup (8 oz.) of whole milk.  The label on a container of whole milk indicates that a cup has 11 grams of

carbohydrate, 8 grams of protein and 9 grams of fat.  The total calories in a cup of whole milk can be determined as follows:

11 gm carbs x 4 Cal per gm =  44 Cal
8 gm protein x 4 Cal per gm = 32 Cal
9 gms fat x 9 Cal per gram =  81 Cal
Total = 44+32+81 = <u>157 Calories</u>

In order to understand the calorie content of a meal, you must be able to estimate both the calorie value of foods as well as portion sizes.  A sense of the **caloric value per ounce** of some <u>basic foods</u> are listed in Table 8.  The extremes of the chart are represented by water the lowest, at zero Calories, and fat (lard) the highest at about 260 Calories per ounce.  Sugar (a pure carbohydrate) is near the middle of the ranking at 110 Calories per ounce .  Protein is also approximately 110 Calories per ounce but there is no pure protein food to rank.  (Note, most of the calorie per ounce values in Table 8 are the average of many varieties in a particular category.)

| **Water** | **0** | Pasta | 36 |
|---|---|---|---|
| Coffee or Tea | 1 | Fish | 42 |
| Vegetables | 7 | Eggs | 47 |
| Milk (fat free) | 10 | Poultry | 54 |
| Soft drink | 12 | Whiskey | 71 |
| Beer | 13 | Bread | 72 |
| Fruit | 15 | Meat | 97 |
| Milk (whole) | 18 | Cake | 100 |
| Potato | 23 | **Sugar** | **110** |
| Corn | 25 | Chocolate | 151 |
| Wine | 27 | Nuts | 175 |
| Rice | 33 | Vegetable oil | 253 |
| Beans | 34 | **Lard** | **260** |

**Table 8: Calorie Rank of Basic Foods**

| Food | Cal | Food | Cal | Food | Cal |
|---|---|---|---|---|---|
| **Water** | **0** | Peas | 20 | Liverwurst | 79 |
| Coffee or Tea | 1 | Yogurt (whole) | 21 | Hamburger | 82 |
| Vinegar | 3 | Potato (boiled) | 23 | Tuna (in oil) | 82 |
| Lettuce | 4 | Clams (raw) | 25 | Raisins | 83 |
| Celery | 5 | Banana | 25 | Bologna | 87 |
| Asparagus | 6 | Corn | 25 | Wheat Flakes | 89 |
| Tomato | 7 | Wine | 27 | Cake (average) | 100 |
| Spinach | 7 | Lobster | 27 | Sirloin Steak | 103 |
| Watermelon | 7 | Lentils | 30 | Cheese | 106 |
| Lemon | 8 | Scallops | 32 | Ham (baked) | 106 |
| Broccoli | 8 | Rice | 33 | Oatmeal | 107 |
| Mushrooms | 9 | Beans | 34 | **Sugar** | **110** |
| Cantaloupe | 10 | Pasta | 36 | Pretzels | 111 |
| Milk (fat free) | 10 | Tuna (in water) | 36 | Crackers | 114 |
| Carrots | 10 | Olives (black) | 37 | Doughnut | 117 |
| Strawberries | 11 | Blue Fish (baked) | 45 | Fudge | 117 |
| Green Pepper | 11 | Egg (boiled) | 47 | Chocolate | 151 |
| Peach | 11 | Turkey (light) | 50 | Potato Chips | 162 |
| Grapefruit | 11 | Ice Cream | 55 | Peanut Butter | 167 |
| Cola Drink | 12 | Sardines | 56 | Almonds | 171 |
| Beer | 13 | Turkey (dark) | 58 | Bacon | 175 |
| Yogurt (fat free) | 13 | Pancakes | 64 | Walnuts | 180 |
| Orange | 14 | Bread (wheat) | 69 | Butter | 205 |
| Apple | 16 | Whisky-86 proof | 71 | Mayonnaise | 205 |
| Milk (whole) | 18 | Apple Pie | 73 | Margarine | 206 |
| Cherries | 19 | Bread (white) | 77 | Vegetable Oil | 253 |
| Grapes | 19 | Jam/Jelly | 78 | **Lard (fat)** | **260** |

**Table 10: Calorie Rank of Common Foods**

Table 9 is an expanded version of the Table 8 that includes the **Calories per ounce** of some commonly encountered foods.

If you appreciate that **most foods are some combination of water,**

**carbs, protein, fat and fiber**, this can lead to a better understanding of why a particular food has the caloric value and rank shown in Table 9. For example, watermelon is almost entirely water, with some fiber (zero calories) and carbohydrate, with no protein or fat, and consequently has a very low 7 Calories per ounce value. A grape is again mostly water with some fiber and carbohydrate and according to the chart has only 19 Calories per ounce, but a raisin (a dried grape) is almost entirely carbohydrate and fiber with little water and thus has a value of 83 Calories per ounce – closer to the 110 Calories per ounce of a pure carbohydrate. When a food is not listed in the chart, common sense can often be used to estimate its caloric value; e.g., green beans are not listed, but judging from the ranking of similar foods a value of 6 or 7 Calories per ounce seems reasonable.

Table 9 can also be thought of as a listing of the "caloric density" of foods. For instance, the table illustrates that eight ounces (half pound) of carrots contains about 80 Calories, or approximately the same number of calories as one ounce of hamburger at 82 Calories per ounce. (Note that the numbers in the table are approximate Calories per fluid or dry ounce.)

Moreover, Table 9 in combination with a small weighing scale makes a very useful diet aide, allowing the calorie value of many food portions to be estimated quite accurately. It is a simple mater to weigh a piece of meat or a pancake, or a slice of apple pie, and multiply the weight in ounces by the calorie value per ounce (from Table 9) to determine the total number of calories. Frequently, this approach will result in more precise calorie values than those obtained from the numbers shown in a common calorie table where the portion size is often ambiguously described.

## Common-Sense Nutrition

**1) Know your daily weight maintenance caloric allowance** (More about this later.).

**2) Eat a variety of foods** within your caloric allowance, and consult the **Basic Food Groups** on page 42 to shape your eating patterns. Try to choose the proper quantity from each food group.

**3) Try not to consume foods containing partially-hydrogenated vegetable oil** because they are high in trans fats. This includes commercially prepared baked goods, snack foods, and processed foods, including most fast foods.

**4) Limit your intake of saturated fats.** Eat meat less often and fish and poultry more often, and use fat-free milk and milk products.

**5) When possible, select fresh and natural foods and whole-grain products,** and avoid chemical preservatives and additives, artificial and imitation foods, refined and processed foods, and foods that are mostly "nutritionally-empty calories."

6) **Eat nutritionally-dense foods** rather than calorie-dense foods.
7) **Take a daily multi-vitamin/mineral supplement.**
8) Before you buy, **read and understand the labels on food packages.**

## Eat Slowly

One final important point, try to **eat slowly**.  This is especially vital if you are on a diet, trying to lose weight.  If you are someone who eats fast, who finishes before everyone else at the table, you are not giving yourself a chance to feel full.  While everyone else is still eating, you either sit there and pick, or you have seconds, taking in extra calories you could avoid if you would just slow down.  To slow down, try eating smaller mouthfuls, try chewing your food more thoroughly, and try talking more at the table.

## Further Information

For more information on other important nutrition topics such as purchasing food, storing food and preparing food see USDA Home and Garden Bulletin No. 1.  This publication is somewhat outdated but is still a very good guide and contains a great deal of useful data – all in one document.  At this writing the bulletin  is available free of charge on the internet.

# 5. LIFE-LONG NUTRITION

There are lots of reasons to practice good nutrition: a longer life expectancy, less illness, a healthful appearance, and more energy for daily living. In short, you will be healthier, feel better and look better too!

Why then is it so easy to become a dropout when healthy eating offers such wonderful benefits? A plan may be the missing link. Many in the health profession believe that it is especially **important for an individual starting a healthy eating program to set goals, have a plan and keep a log of what they eat.**

## Have a Plan - Keep a Log

Everyone's personal goals and plan of attack will be different. Let us assume your goals are to improve your overall health and lose weight. First, commit yourself and start immediately. (Buy a notebook, use your laptop, or your Smart Phone because you will need to put your goals and plans in writing.)

Next, plan how you are going to attain these goals. Broadly speaking, your overall plan might be to start eating healthier foods and to begin a weight loss diet. You must, however, be more specific and develop a detailed plan that indicates the when and how you are going to start eating healthier foods, how much weight you want to lose, etcetera. Note the date you plan to start and milestone dates. Put it in writing!

First start a log of what you are currently eating. Then edit the log by making changes to reflect how you are going to eat in the future. For example if your usual breakfast consists of a donut and diet coke, edit this to a more nutritious glass of juice, bowl of cereal with skim milk and fruit.

For the weight loss portion of your plan, decide if you are going to go it alone or join some sort of clinical or non-clinical program. [Incidentally, all the information you need for a do-it-yourself weight loss program can be found in *Weight Control - U.S. Edition* by Vincent Antonetti, Ph.D., published by NoPaperPress.] If you settle on a do-it-yourself program, note the diet calorie level, milestone dates for weight loss, etcetera. Put it in writing!

By now you must appreciate why you need a notebook. As you progress, periodically update your fitness plan. Enlist the support of your family and friends and do not forget to reward yourself when you reach a milestone – for a job well done!

## Exercise is Important

In many developed countries, the general lack of fitness of countless adults, who begin to show signs of old age – shortness of breath, obesity and clogged arteries – years earlier than their counterparts of just a few generations ago, is considered a national problem.

So if you are not getting enough exercise, this would be a perfect time to include exercise into your healthier living program. Assuming you have medical clearance, most fitness experts recommend that you engage in some form of moderate aerobic exercise every single day of the year. That is right every day! And also get in some moderate strength training at least two non-consecutive days per week. [For more information see *Total Fitness - U.S. Edition* also published by NoPaperPress.]

## Summarize Your Nutritional Needs

It's a good idea to summarize your daily nutritional needs. That way you'll have in one place the number of calories, and the nutrient and micronutrient amounts you should be eating on a daily basis.. How to go about accomplishing this is again best illustrated by an example.

**Example:** Summarize the daily nutritional needs of a healthy 45-year old, 5'-11", 180-pound male who describes himself as moderately active. He is in weight maintenance mode.

This person's nutritional needs include his maintenance calories [which can be found in either *Total Fitness - U.S. Edition* or *Weight Control - U.S. Edition* - both published by NoPaperPress], the amount of protein and fat grams he should consume, and the micronutrient (vitamin and mineral) requirements specific to his age and gender. All this and more is shown in Table 10.

For each line, there is an amount, the basis for the amount, and the food source - all documented. For instance, the entry for vitamin A lists the amount (RDA) as 900 mcg; the basis as Table 10, and the food sources as orange-colored fruit and vegetables. Please note that the cited food sources are what this particular 45-year old man selected based on his specific needs and dietary habits. (In our opinion his choices lack plant-based protein foods such as beans and soy.)

For easy reference, make a chart similar to Table 10 for yourself and put on your refrigerator door, or better yet carry it with you in your briefcase, on your Smart Phone, laptop, or whatever works for you.

|  | **Amount** | **Basis** | **Food Source & notes** |
|---|---|---|---|
| **Weight** (lbs) | 183 | --- | From example |
| **Total Calories** | 2,975 | --- | *Weight Control - US Edition* |
| **Protein** | 66 g | 0.36 g/lb | --- |
| **Max Total Fat** | 99 g | 30% of calories | Fat gm = Cal divided by 9 |
| **Max Sat Fat** | 33 g | 10% of calories | Fat gm = Cal divided by 9 |
| **Omega-3** (g) | -- | --- | Fish 2 to 3 times per week |
| **Fiber** | 25 g | --- | Cereal, bread & veggies |
| **A** (mcg) | 900 | Table 5 | Orange-colored fruit/veggies |
| **D** (mcg) | 5 | Table 5 | Milk & yogurt |
| **E** (mcg) | 15 | Table 5 | Nuts & seeds |
| **K** (mcg)* | 120 | Table 5 | Balanced diet |
| **C** (mg) | 90 | Table 5 | 6 oz orange juice |
| **B$_1$** (mg) | 1.2 | Table 5 | Fortified cereal |
| **B$_2$** (mg) | 1.3 | Table 5 | Fortified cereal |
| **B$_3$** (mg) | 16 | Table 5 | Fortified cereal |
| **B$_5$** (mg) | 5 | Table 5 | Fortified cereal |
| **B$_6$** (mg) | 1.3 | Table 5 | Fortified cereal |
| **B$_7$** (mcg) | 30 | Table 5 | Vitamin/mineral supplement |
| **B$_9$** (mcg) | 400 | Table 5 | Fortified cereal |
| **B$_{12}$** (mcg) | 2.4 | Table 5 | Fortified cereal |
| **Calcium** (mg) | 1000 | Table 6 | Milk & dark-green veggies |
| **Chromium** (mcg) | 35 | Table 6 | Fortified cereal & peanut |
| **Copper** (mcg) | 900 | Table 6 | Vitamin/mineral supplement |
| **Fluoride** (mg) | 4 | Table 6 | Fluorinated water |
| **Iodine** (mcg) | 150 | Table 6 | Fish 2 to 3 times per week |
| **Iron** (mg) | 8 | Table 6 | Fortified cereal |
| **Magnesium** (mg) | 420 | Table 6 | Dark-green-leafy vegetables |
| **Manganese** (mg) | 2.3 | Table 6 | Vitamin/mineral supplement |
| **Molybdenum** | 45 | Table 6 | Vitamin/mineral supplement |
| **Phosphorus** (mg) | 700 | Table 6 | Milk, yogurt & fish |
| **Potassium** (mg) | 4700 | Table 6 | Bananas, oranges & leafy |
| **Selenium** (mcg) | 55 | Table 6 | Fish 2 to 3 times per week |
| **Zinc** (mg) | 11 | Table 6 | Fortified cereal |

**Table 11: Nutritional Needs of Man in Example**

## Now It's Up To You

At this point, you have everything you need to succeed. You have an understanding of the fundamentals of nutrition. You have set realistic goals, and you have a good plan. If you combine all these with intense desire you'll be unstoppable. Your new nutritional regimen will work wonders and will have you looking and feeling better both physically and mentally. And when you look and feel your best, your spirit will soar. So as you start on the road to better health, be aware that you are well prepared for success and always keep in mind how good you'll feel when you reach your goals.

# BIBLIOGRAPHY

A Primer on Fats and Oils. ADA website accessed July 2004, http://www.eatright.org

Antonetti, V.W. *Total Fitness - U.S. Edition*. eBook and paperback published by NoPaperPress, 2006.

Antonetti, V.W. *Total Weight Control - U.S. Edition*. eBook published by NoPaperPress, 2006.

Bennion, M. and Scheule, B. *Introductory Foods*. Prentice-Hall, Upper Saddle River, NJ, 2000.

Biong, A.S., Veierød, M.B., Ringstad, J., Thelle, D.S. and Pedersen, J.I. Intake of milk fat, reflected in adipose tissue fatty acids and risk of myocardial infarction: a case–control study. *Eur J Clin Nutr* 2005;60:236-244.

Cao, G., et al. Increases in human plasma antioxidant capacity after consumption of controlled diets high in fruit and vegetables. *Am J Clin Nutr* 1998;68:1081-1087.

Fleet, J.C. DASH without the dash (of salt) can lower blood pressure. *Nutr Rev* 2001;59(9): 291-297.

Coleman, E. and Steen, S.N. *The Ultimate Sports Nutrition Handbook*. Bull Publishing, Palo Alto, CA, 1996.

Consumers Union. Is a multivitamin enough? Too much? *Consumer Reports Onhealth* 2004;16(10)1, 4-6.

Cashel, K., English, R. and Lewis, J. eds., *Composition of Foods*, Australia (5 manuals),
Australian Government Publishing Service, 1989.

de Lorgeril M., et al. Mediterranean diet, traditional risk factors, and the rate of cardiovascular complications after myocardial infarction: Final report of the Lyon Diet Heart Study, *Circulation* 1999;99:779-785

Dietary Guidelines for Americans, 2005. U.S. Government Printing Office No. 001-000-04719-1.
http://www.health.gov/dietaryguidelines/dga2000/document/build.htm

Dixon, L.B., et al. Choose a diet that is low in saturated fat and cholesterol and moderate in total fat:subtle changes to a familiar message. *J Nutr* 2001;131:510S-526S.

Duggan, C., et al. Protective nutrients and functional foods for the gastrointestinal tract. *Am J Clin Nutr* 2002;75(5):789-808.

Duyff, R.L. *American Dietetic Association Complete Food and Nutrition Guide*, 2nd edition. John Wiley & Sons, Hoboken, NJ, 2002.

Edwards, A.J., et al. Consumption of watermelon juice increases plasma concentrations of lycopene and beta-carotene in humans. *J Nutr* 2003;133(4):1043-1050.

Erlund, I., et al. Consumption of black currants, lingonberries and bilberries increases serum quercetin concentrations. *Eur J Clin Nutr* 2003;57(1)37-42.

Feldman, E.B., The scientific evidence for a beneficial health relationship between walnuts and coronary heart disease. *J Nutr* 2002;132(5):1062S-1101S.

Fraser, G.E., et al. Risk factors for all-cause and coronary heart disease mortality in the oldest-old. The Adventist Health Study. *Arch Intern Med* 1997;157:2249-2258.

Gebhardt, S. E. and Thomas, R. G. *Nutritive Value of Foods*, USDA. Home and Garden Bulletin No. 72: 2002.

Geleijnse, J.M., et al. Inverse association of tea and flavonoids intakes with incident myocardial infarction: the Rotterdam Study. *Am J Clin Nutr* 2002:75;880-886.

Guidelines for Healthy Aerobic Activity and Calculating Your Exercise Heart Rate Range. American College of Sports Medicine website accessed October 2006, http://www.acsm.org/health+fitness/index.htm

Hadley, C.W., et al. The consumption of processed tomato products enhances plasma lycopene concentrations in association with reduced lipoprotein sensitivity to oxidative damage. *J Nutr* 2003;133(3):727-732.

Herbert, V. and Subak, G.J.,eds *Total Nutrition: The Only Guide You'll Ever Need - From The Mount Sinai School Of Medicine*.  St. Martin's Griffin, New York, 1995.

Carbohydrates. Harvard School of Public Health website accessed December 2005. http://www.hsph.harvard.edu/nutrionsource/

Hertog, M.G., et al. Antioxidant flavonols and coronary heart disease risk. *Lancet* 1997:349.

Hites, R.A., et al. Global Assessment of Organic Contaminants in Farmed Salmon. *Science*. 2004:303 (5655):226-229.

Hole, J.W. *Human Anatomy and Physiology*. Wm. C. Brown, Dubuque, IA, 1978.

Hu, F.B.,et al. A prospective study of egg consumption and risk of cardiovascular disease in men and women. *JAMA* 1999;281(15):1387-1394.

Institute of Medicine. *Dietary Reference Intakes for Energy, Carbohydrate, Fiber, Fat, Fatty Acids, Cholesterol, Protein, and Amino Acids*. Nat Academy Press. Washington, DC, 2002.

Johnston, L., et al. Cholesterol-lowering benefits of a whole grain ready-to-eat oat cereal. *Nutr Clin Care* 1998;1:6-12.

Johnston, C.S., et al. Stability of ascorbic acid in commercially available orange juices. *J Am Diet Assoc* 2002;102:525-529.

Kant, A.K., et al. Dietary diversity and subsequent mortality in the first national health and nutrition survey epidemiologic follow-up study. *Am J Clin Nutr* 1993;57:443-440.

Kohlmeier, L., et al. Epidemiologic evidence of a role of carotenoids in cardiovascular disease prevention. *Am J Clin Nutr* 1995;62:1370S-1368S.

Krebs-Smith, S.M., et al. The effects of variety in food choices on dietary quality. *J Am Diet Assoc* 1987;87(7):896-902.

Kris-Etherton P. Fish consumption, fish oil, omega-3 fatty acids, and cardiovascular disease. AHA Scientific Statement, *Circulation* 2002;106:2747-2757.

Kushi, L.H., et al. Cereals, legumes, and chronic disease risk reduction: evidence from epidemiologic studies. *Am J Clin Nutr* 1999;70:451S-458S.

Levine, M., et al. Criteria and recommendations for vitamin C intake. *JAMA* 1999;281:1415-1423.

Marlett, J.A., et al. Position of the American Dietetic Association: health implications of dietary fiber. *J Am Diet Assoc* 2002;102(7):993-1000.

Messina, M. Legumes and soybeans: overview of their nutritional profiles and health effects. *Am J Clin Nutr* 1999;70:439S-450S.

Miller, H.E., et al. Antioxidant content of whole grain breakfast cereals, fruits and vegetables. *J Am Coll Nutr* 2000;19:312S-319S.

Monroe, I.C., et al. Soy isoflavones: a safety review. *Nutr Rev* 2003;61(1):1-33.

Nestle, M. Broccoli sprouts in cancer prevention. *Nutr Rev* 1998;56(pt 1):127-130.

Pitsavos, C., et al. Adherence to the Mediterranean diet is associated with total antioxidant capacity in healthy adults: the ATTICA study. *Am J Clin Nutr* 2005;82(3): 694-699.

President's Council on Physical Fitness & Sports website accessed on April 2006, http://fitness.gov/council_pubs.htm

Ramakrishnan, U. Prevalence of micronutrient malnutrition worldwide. *Nutr Rev* 2002;60(5, PartII): S46-S52.

Rimm, E.B., et al. Vegetable, fruit, and cereal fiber intake and risk of coronary heart disease. *JAMA* 1996;275:447-451.

Simopoulos, A.P. Essential fatty acids in health and chronic disease. Am J Clin Nutr 1999:70:56S-59S.

Slavin, J., et al. Plausible mechanisms for the protectiveness of whole grains. *Am J Clin Nutr* 1999;70:459-463S.

State of World Fisheries and Aquaculture. United Nations FAO (Food and Agricultural Organization). 2004, Green Facts website accessed February 2006, http://www.greenfacts.org/fisheries/about-fisheries.htm#1

Tidow-Kebritchi, S., et al. Effects of diets containing fish oil and vitamin E on rheumatoid arthritis. *Nutr Rev* 2001;59:335-337.

Ulene, A. *The NutriBase Nutrition Facts Desk Reference*. Garden City Park, NY: Avery Publishing Group, 1995.

University of Sydney Glycemic Database. Website accessed December 2006. http://www.glycemicindex.com/

USDA National Nutrient Database for Standard Reference. USDA Nutrient Data Laboratory, accessed December 2004. http://www.nal.usda.gov/fnic/foodcomp/search/

USDA Nutrient List.  Nutrition.gov web site accessed October 2006, http://www.nutrition.gov/

USDA Home & Garden Bulletin No. 1 Family Fare – A guide to good nutrition, 1978.

Willcox, B.J., et al. *The Okinawa Program*, Three Rivers Press, New York, 2001.

Willet, W.C. *Eat, Drink and Be Healthy - The Harvard Medical School Guide to Healthy Eating*. Simon & Schuster. New York, 2001.

Willmore, J.H. and Costill, D.L. *Physiology of Sport and Exercise*, 3rd ed.. Human Kinetics Publishers, Champaign, IL, 2004.

Wing, R.R. and Phelan, S. Long-term weight loss maintenance. Am J Clin Nutr  2005;82:222S-225S.

Wise, J.A. *Health benefits of fruits and vegetables: the protective role of phytonutrients. Vegetables, Fruits and Herbs in Health Promotion*. Watson, R.R. ed. CRC Press: 2001;147-76.

## Disclaimer

This book offers general nutrition information. It is not a medical manual and the author does not claim to be medically qualified. The material in this book is not intended to be a substitute for medical counseling. Everyone should have a medical checkup before making major changes to their eating patterns. This is particularly important for anyone with medical problems and for women who are pregnant or breast-feeding, all of whom should consult a physician or registered dietician to determine the dietary pattern that is appropriate for them. Moreover, the physician conducting the medical exam should be made aware of and should approve the specific nutritional changes planned. Additionally, while the author and publisher have made every effort to ensure the accuracy of the information in this book, they make no representations or warranties regarding its accuracy or completeness. Neither the author nor publisher assume liability for any medical problems that might result from applying the methods in this book, or for any loss of profit, or any other commercial damages, including but not limited to special, incidental, consequential or other damages, and any such liability is hereby expressly disclaimed.

# <u>NoPaperPress eBooks and Paperbacks</u>

100-Day Super Diet-1200 Cal*
100-Day Super Diet-1500 Cal*
100-Day No-Cooking Diet-1200 Cal*
100-Day No-Cooking Diet-1500 Cal*
90-Day Smart Diet-1200 Cal*
90-Day Smart Diet-1500 Cal*
90-Day No-Cooking Diet - 1200 Cal*
90-Day No-Cooking Diet - 1500 Cal*
90-Day Perfect Diet - 1200 Cal*
90-Day Perfect Diet - 1500 Cal*
60-Day Perfect Diet-1200 Cal*
60-Day Perfect Diet-1500 Cal*
50-Day Flex Diet-1200 Cal*
50-Day Flex Diet-1500 Cal*
30-Day Quick Diet - Women*
30-Day Quick Diet for Men*
30-Day No-Cooking Diet*
30-Day Diet - Women - Metric*
30-Day Diet for Men - Metric*
25 Day Easy Diet-1200 Cal*
25 Day Easy Diet-1500 Cal*
25-Day No-Cooking Diet
10-Day Express Diet
10-Day No-Cooking Diet*
7-Day Diet for Women*
7-Day Diet for Men*
7-Day No-Cooking Diets*
90-Day Gluten-Free Diet-1200 Cal*
90-Day Gluten-Free Diet-1500 Cal*
30-Day Gluten-Free Quick Diet*
30-Day Gluten-Free No-Cooking Diet*
7-Day Diet for Women - Metric*
7-Day Diet for Men - Metric
7-Day Gluten-Free Express Diet*
7-Day Gluten-Free No-Cooking Diet*
90-Day Vegetarian Diet-1200 Cal*
90-Day Vegetarian Diet-1500 Cal*
30-Day Vegetarian Diet*
7-Day Vegetarian Diet*
Weight Loss for Women*
Weight Loss for Women - Metric
Weight Loss for Women - UK
Weight Loss for Men*
Maximum Weight Loss - 1200 Cal*
Maximum Weight Loss - 1500 Cal*

Weight Loss for Men - Metric*
Maximum Weight Loss- 1200 Cal*
Maximum Weight Loss- 1500 Cal*
Weight Control - U.S. Edition*
Weight Control - Metric. Edition
Prof Weight Control Women - U.S.
Prof Weight Control Women - Metric
Prof Weight Control Men - U.S.
Prof Weight Control Men - Metric
Weight Maintenance - U.S. Ed*
Weight Maintenance - Metric. Ed*
Weight Maintenance - UK Ed
Weight Loss for Senior Men*
Weight Loss for Senior Women*
Eat Smart - U.S. Edition*
Eat Smart - Metric Edition
30-Day Mediterranean Diet
Exercise Smart - U.S. Edition*
Exercise Smart - Metric Edition
Exercise Smart - UK Edition*
Total Fitness - U.S. Edition
Total Fitness - Metric Edition
Total Fitness - UK Edition
Total Fitness for Women-U.S. Ed*
Total Fitness for Women - Metric
Total Fitness for Women - UK Ed
Total Fitness for Men - U.S. Ed*
Total Fitness for Men- Metric Ed*
Total Fitness for Men - UK Ed
Senior Fitness - U.S. Edition*
Senior Fitness - Metric Edition*
Senior Fitness - UK Edition*
Computer Diet - U.S. Edition*
Computer Diet - Metric Ed*
Reliable Weight Loss - U.S. Ed
101 Weight Loss Tips*
101 Healthy Eating Tips*
101 Lifelong Fitness Tips*
101 Weight Maintenance Tips
101 Weight Loss Recipes
101 GF Weight Loss Recipes
101 Veggie Weight Loss Recipes*
30-Day Mediterranean Diet*
90-Day Mediterranean Diet - 1200 Cal*
90-Day Mediterranean Diet - 1500 Cal*

* These titles are available as both ebooks and paperbacks. Our ebooks are sold by Amazon, Apple, Google, Barnes & Noble and Kobo, but our paperbacks are only sold by Amazon.